MW00604518

The
Nursing
Assistant's
Handbook

By Hartman Publishing, Inc.
with Jetta Fuzy, RN, MS

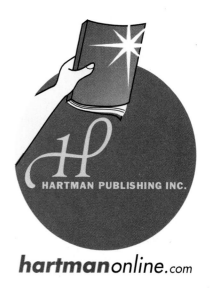

HARTMAN PUBLISHING INC.

*hartman*online.com

Credits

MANAGING EDITOR
Susan Alvare

COVER AND INTERIOR DESIGNER
Kirsten Browne

ILLUSTRATORS
Thaddeus Castillo/Robert Christopher

PAGE LAYOUT
Thaddeus Castillo

PHOTOGRAPHY
Art Clifton/Dick Ruddy/Susanita Marcos

NURSE CONSULTANT
Bonnie Neorr, RN

PROOFREADERS
Kristin Dyche
Joey Tulino/Yvonne Gillam

SALES/MARKETING
Gailynn Garberding/Yvonne Gillam

CUSTOMER SERVICE
Lea Collinet

Copyright Information

NOTICE TO READERS
Though the guidelines and procedures contained in this text are based on consultations with healthcare professionals, they should not be considered absolute recommendations. The instructor and readers should follow employer, local, state, and federal guidelines concerning healthcare practices. These guidelines change, and it is the reader's responsibility to be aware of these changes and of the policies and procedures of her or his healthcare facility.

The publisher, author, editors, and reviewers cannot accept any responsibility for errors or omissions or for any consequences from application of the information in this book and make no warranty, expressed or implied, with respect to the contents of the book. The Publisher does not warrant or guarantee any of the products described herein or perform any analysis in connection with any of the product information contained herein.

GENDER USAGE
This textbook utilizes the pronouns he, his, she, and hers interchangeably to denote healthcare team members and residents.

Special Thanks

We are so appreciative of our insightful and always available reviewers:

Bonnie Neorr, RN

Marianna Kern Grachek, MSN, CNHA, CALA

Clara McElroy, RN, MA, LMT

Ruth Hardke-Peck, LPN, SDC

Diane Crooks, LVN

Cheryl Dilbeck, MN, RN, PHN, NEC

Katherine Purgatorio Howard, MS, RN, BC

Loretta Tillman, RN

Joanne Baty, RN, MA

Linda Bolick, RN

Gloria Kas, RN, BS

Jessica Schwipps, LPN

A heartfelt thank you to Sarah Harris, RN, who served as our technical advisor on the photo shoot.

We are grateful for our beautiful and agreeable models who worked on our most recent photo shoot: Lorene Ervin, Yvonne Gillam, Mark Hartman, and Sarah Harris.

We extend a special thank you to Ryan Martino for his expertise and ability to meet tough deadlines.

Many wonderful and informative photos came from the following sources:
Lee Penner of Penner Tubs
The Briggs Corporation
Northcoast Medical, Inc.
Innovative Products Unlimited
Dr. Frederick Miller
Dr. Jeffrey T. Behr
VANCARE, Inc.
Merry Walker Corporation

TABLE OF CONTENTS

𝓟 denotes a practical procedure

WELCOME TO
The Nursing
Assistant's
HANDBOOK!

We have divided this book into ten chapters and assigned each chapter its own colored tab, which you'll see on the side of every page. At the top of every page, you'll find the name of the section that is being taught.

Unit 1. Describe the integumentary system

Everything you will learn in this book is organized around learning objectives. A learning objective is a specific piece of knowledge or a very specific skill.

All care procedures will have numbered steps. Underneath each step is the reason why it is important for you to perform this step.

This sign shows you how specific information relates to the study of the human body.

This icon is found at the end of some procedures. It points out common errors that students make when they are tested on this skill during a certification exam.

This icon emphasizes Residents' Rights. These are very important rights for residents who live in nursing homes. They are the law and must always be followed.

State agencies perform inspections on nursing homes on a regular basis. These inspections are called surveys. This sign shows you what facilities are often cited for during surveys.

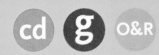

You'll find bold **key terms** throughout the text. These are important terms you need to know. COMMON DISORDERS, GUIDELINES, and OBSERVING AND REPORTING are also colored for easy reference.

ONE

Long-Term Care and the Nursing Assistant's Role

Unit 1: **Compare long-term care to other healthcare settings**

Unit 2: **Describe a typical long-term care facility**

Unit 3: **Explain Medicare and Medicaid**

Unit 4: **Describe the role of the nursing assistant**

Unit 5: **Describe the care team and the chain of command**

Unit 6: **Define policies, procedures and professionalism**

Unit 7: **List examples of legal and ethical behavior and explain residents' rights**

Unit 8: **Explain legal aspects of the resident's medical record**

Unit 1: Compare long-term care to other healthcare settings

Welcome to the world of health care. Health care happens in many types of places. Nursing assistants work in many of these settings. In each setting, similar tasks will be performed. However, each setting is also unique in some ways.

Some of the settings include the following:

Acute care is performed in hospitals and ambulatory surgical centers. Persons are admitted for short stays for surgery or diseases. Acute care offers 24-hour skilled care for temporary, but serious, illnesses or injuries (Fig. 1-1).

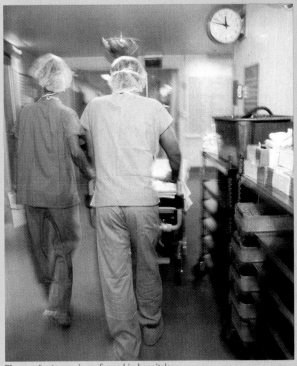

Fig. 1-1. Acute care is performed in hospitals.

Subacute care can be found in either a hospital or a traditional nursing home. The residents need more daily care and observation than a long-term care facility can offer. The cost for these services is usually less than a hospital but more than long-term care.

Outpatient care is usually provided for less than 24-hours for persons who have had treatments or surgery that require short-term skilled care.

Rehabilitation is care provided by a specialist. This is a person trained to provide special care. Physical, occupational, and speech therapists restore or improve a resident's function after an illness or injury.

Home care is provided in a person's home. Home care includes many of the services offered in other settings (Fig. 1-2).

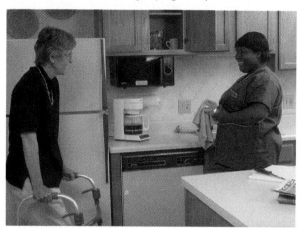

Fig. 1-2. Home care is performed in a person's home.

In **assisted living** residents need some assistance with daily care, such as showers and meals. They may also need assistance with medications. They do not usually require skilled care.

Hospice care is for individuals who have six months or less to live. Hospice provides physical and emotional care and comfort. It also supports families. Hospice care can take place in facilities or in private homes.

Long-term care (LTC) is for persons who require 24-hour care and assistance for conditions that are long-term. Other terms used for long-term care include nursing homes, nursing facility, skilled nursing facility, or extended care facility. The people who live here may be disabled and/or elderly. They may come from hospitals or other facilities. Some people will have a terminal illness. **Terminal** means the person will die with the illness. Other people come to nursing homes for conditions that require care for six months or longer. Some of these persons recover and return to their homes or to assisted living facilities. Most conditions seen in nursing homes are **chronic**. This means they last a long period of time, even over a lifetime. Chronic conditions include physical disabilities, heart disease, stroke, and dementia. (You will learn more about these disorders and diseases in chapter 8.) Working in a nursing home, you will form relationships with residents for longer periods of time than in other healthcare settings.

The person for whom you will care may be called a resident, patient, or client. The person's **diagnosis**, or medical condition, will differ from one setting to another. The stages of illnesses or diseases affect how sick people are and how much care they will need. The job of the nursing assistant who works in these settings will also vary. This is due to the person's different symptoms, abilities, and needs. This book will focus on the role of the nursing assistant in the nursing home. The people who live in nursing homes are called **residents**. This is how this book will refer to the people for whom you will be providing care.

Unit 2: **Describe a typical long-term care facility**

A long-term care facility may provide only

skilled nursing care. It may also offer assisted living, dementia care, or even subacute care. Some facilities specialize in certain types of residents. Others provide care for all types of residents. The typical long-term care facility offers personal care for all residents and focused care for residents with special needs. When specialized care is offered, the employees may have special training. Residents with similar conditions may be placed in units or wings together.

The organization of most long-term care facilities is the same as that of other healthcare settings. For-profit companies or nonprofit organizations can own them. More information about the care team and how the members work together is provided later in the chapter.

Unit 3: **Explain Medicare and Medicaid**

The Centers for Medicare & Medicaid Services (CMS), formerly the Health Care Finance Administration (HCFA), is a federal agency within the U.S. Department of Health and Human Services. CMS runs two national healthcare programs, Medicare and Medicaid. They both help pay for health care and health insurance for millions of Americans.

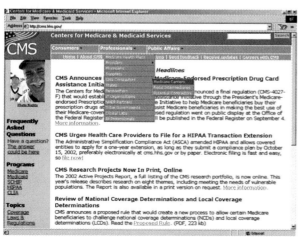

Fig. 1-3. The CMS web site.

Medicare is a health insurance program for people over 65 years old. It also covers people younger than 65 but who are disabled and unable to work. Medicare has a Part A and a Part B, which cover different medical services. Medicare covers a percentage of a person's healthcare costs.

Medicaid is a medical assistance program for low-income people. The coverage is limited, and a person has to qualify to receive it.

Medicare and Medicaid pay long-term care facilities a fixed amount for services for residents. This is based on the resident's need upon admission.

Unit 4: **Describe the role of the nursing assistant**

Nursing assistants can have many different titles. Nurse aide, unlicensed assistive personnel, and certified nursing assistant are some examples. This book will use the term "nursing assistant." The nursing assistant (NA) performs delegated or assigned nursing tasks, such as taking someone's temperature. A nursing assistant also provides personal care, such as bathing residents.

Other nursing assistant duties include

- feeding residents
- helping residents with toileting and elimination needs
- assisting residents to move safely around the facility
- keeping residents' living areas neat and clean
- encouraging residents to eat and drink (Fig. 1-4)
- caring for supplies and equipment
- helping dress residents
- making beds

Long-Term Care and the Nursing Assistant's Role

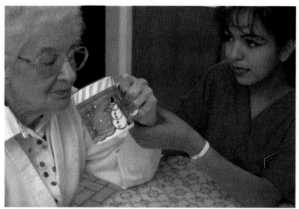

Fig. 1-4. Assisting a resident with drinking will be one of your duties.

- giving back massages
- assisting residents with mouth care

📋 *Nursing assistants are not allowed to give medications. Nurses are responsible for giving medications. Some states allow nursing assistants to give medications under certain conditions after receiving additional training.*

Nursing assistants spend more time with residents than other members of the health-care team. They act as the "eyes and ears" of the team. Observing changes in a resident's condition and reporting them to other team members is a very important role. In addition, you will write down important information about the resident (Fig. 1-5). Writing down information is called **charting**.

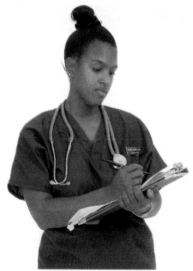

Fig. 1-5. Writing down your observations is one of the most important duties you'll have.

Nursing assistants are part of a team of health professionals. The team includes physicians, nurses, social workers, therapists, dietitians, and specialists. The resident's family is part of the team. Everyone, including the resident, works closely together. Goals include helping residents recover from illnesses or to do as much as possible for themselves.

Unit 5: Describe the care team and the chain of command

Because residents have different needs and problems, professionals with different kinds of education and experience will help care for them (Fig. 1-6). Members of the health-care team may include the following:

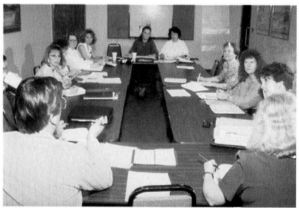

Fig. 1-6. The care team is made up of many different professionals.

Registered Nurse (RN). An RN is a licensed professional who has completed two to four years of education. The nurse in long-term care has two important roles. The first role is to provide skilled nursing care to the resident, including a care plan. A **care plan** is developed for each resident to achieve certain goals. The second role of the nurse is to develop a nursing assistant care plan for each resident. The nurse assigns tasks and supervises the nursing assistant's daily care of the residents (Fig. 1-7).

Licensed Practical Nurse (LPN) or Licensed Vocational Nurse (LVN). A LPN/LVN is a

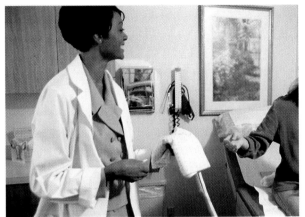
Fig. 1-7. An RN supervises a nursing assistant's care of residents.

licensed professional who has completed one to two years of education. A LPN/LVN passes medications and performs treatments.

Physician (MD). A physician's job is to diagnose disease or disability and prescribe treatment. Physicians have graduated from four-year medical schools, which they attended after receiving a bachelor's degree (Fig. 1-8).

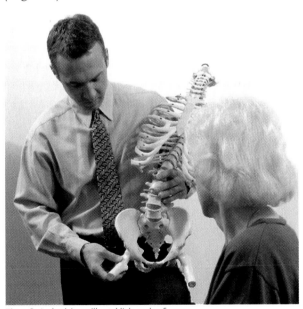
Fig. 1-8. A physician will establish goals of care.

Physical Therapist (PT). The physical therapist administers therapy in the form of heat, cold, massage, ultrasound, electricity, and exercise to muscles, bones, and joints. For example, a physical therapist helps a person to safely use a walker, cane or wheelchair to move from place to place (Fig. 1-9).

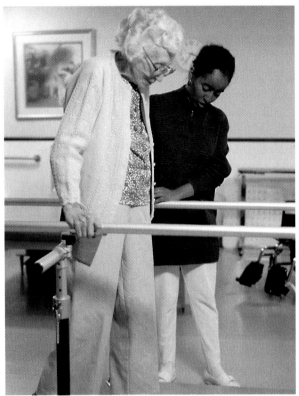
Fig. 1-9. A physical therapist will help restore specific abilities.

Occupational Therapist (OT). An occupational therapist helps residents learn to compensate for disabilities. For example, an occupational therapist teaches a person to use a special spoon so that she can feed herself and remain independent.

Speech Therapist (ST). A speech therapist helps residents with communication. For example, after a stroke, a person may not be able to talk. A speech therapist may use a picture board to have the person communicate thirst or pain. A speech therapist also evaluates a person's ability to swallow food and drink.

Registered Dietitian (RDT). A registered dietitian or nutritionist creates special diets for residents with special needs. Special diets can improve health and help manage illness.

Medical Social Worker (MSW). A medical social worker helps residents with social needs. For example, an MSW helps residents find compatible roommates. An MSW also helps obtain clothing and personal items if the family is not involved or does not visit frequently. An MSW may book dental appointments and arrange transportation.

RA *All members of the healthcare team should focus on the resident. The team revolves around the resident and his or her condition, treatment, and progress. Without the resident, there is no team.*

As a nursing assistant, you are carrying out instructions given to you by a nurse. The nurse is acting on the instructions of a physician or other member of the care team. This is called the **chain of command**. It guarantees that your residents get proper health care. It also protects you and your employer from liability. **Liability** is a legal term that means someone can be held responsible for harming someone else. Example: Something you do for a resident harms him. However, what you did was in the care plan and was done according to policy and procedure. You are not liable, or responsible, for hurting the resident. However, if you do something that is not in the care plan that harms a resident, you could be held responsible. That is why it is important to follow instructions in the care plan and for the facility to have a chain of command (Fig. 1-10).

Nursing assistants must understand what they can and cannot do. This is important so that you do not harm a resident or involve yourself or your employer in a lawsuit. Some states certify that a nursing assistant is qualified to work. However, nursing assistants are not licensed healthcare providers. Everything you do in your job is assigned to you by a licensed healthcare professional. You do your job under the authority of another person's license. That is why these professionals will show great interest in what you do and how you do it.

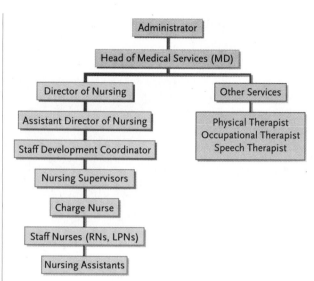

Fig. 1-10. The chain of command ensures that the resident receives the proper care.

Every state grants the right to practice various jobs in health care through licensure. Examples include granting a license to practice nursing, medicine, or physical therapy. All members of the healthcare team work under each professional's "scope of practice." A **scope of practice** defines the things you are allowed to do and how to do them correctly.

Unit 6: **Define policies, procedures and professionalism**

You will be told where to locate the policies and procedures that all staff members are expected to follow. A **policy** is a course of action that should be taken every time a certain situation occurs. For example, one policy at most facilities is that the plan of care must be followed. A **procedure** is a particular method, or way, of doing something. For example, your facility will have a procedure for reporting information about your residents. The procedure tells you what form you fill out, when and how often to fill it out, and to whom it is given.

Common policies at long-term care facilities include the following:

- Information given in a business relationship must remain confidential.

- The resident's plan of care must always be followed.

- Nursing assistants should not do any tasks that are not included in their job description.

- Nursing assistants must report important events or changes in residents to a nurse.

- Personal problems must not be discussed with the resident or the resident's family.

- Nursing assistants must be on time for work and dependable.

Your employer will have policies and procedures for every resident care situation. Though written procedures may seem long and sometimes complicated, each step is important. Become familiar with your facility's policies and procedures.

Professional means having to do with work or a job. The opposite of professional is **personal**, which refers to your life outside your job, such as your family, friends, and home life. **Professionalism** is how you behave when you are on the job. It includes how you dress, the words you use, and the things you talk about. It also includes being on time, completing tasks, and reporting to the nurse. For a nursing assistant, professionalism means following the care plan, being careful to make observations, and always reporting accurately.

Following policies and procedures is an important part of professionalism. Residents, coworkers, and supervisors respect employees who behave in a professional way. Professionalism will help you keep your job and may help you earn promotions and raises.

A professional relationship with a resident includes

- keeping a positive attitude (Fig. 1-11)

- doing only the tasks assigned and ones you are trained to do

- speaking politely and cheerfully to the resident, even if you are not in a good mood

- never discussing any of your personal problems

- calling the resident by the name he or she prefers

- listening to the resident

- always explaining the care you will provide before providing it

- always following care practices, such as handwashing, to protect yourself and the resident

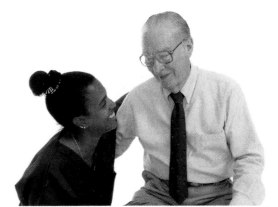

Fig. 1-11. Being polite and cheerful is something that will be expected of you.

A professional relationship with an employer includes

- maintaining a positive attitude

- completing duties efficiently

- consistently following all policies and procedures

- always documenting and reporting carefully and correctly

- communicating problems with residents or duties

- reporting anything that keeps you from

completing duties

- asking questions when you do not know or understand something
- taking directions or criticism without getting upset
- being clean and neatly dressed and groomed (Fig. 1-12)
- always being on time
- notifying your employer if unable to report for work
- following the chain of command
- participating in any education programs offered
- being a positive role model for your facility at all times

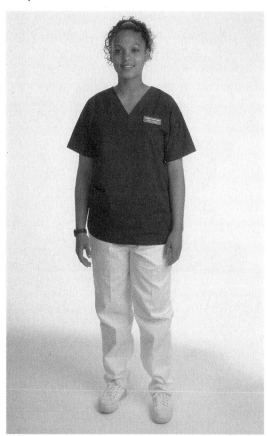

Fig. 1-12. Keeping your hair neatly tied back and wearing a clean uniform are examples of professional behavior.

Qualities of great nursing assistants include being:

- **Compassionate**—caring, concerned, empathetic, and understanding; **empa-thy** means being able to enter into the feelings of others, to put yourself in another person's shoes.
- **Honest**—never saying or doing anything that is not true
- **Conscientious**—always trying to do your best
- **Dependable**—being on time and helping your peers when they need it
- **Respectful**—showing respect for the residents and their belongings
- **Considerate**—being understanding of the residents' feelings and privacy
- **Unprejudiced**—treating all the residents the same regardless of culture, race, religion, or condition
- **Nonjudgmental**—never judging the behavior or conduct of residents

Unit 7: List examples of legal and ethical behavior and explain residents' rights

Ethics and laws guide our behavior. **Ethics** is the knowledge of right and wrong. An ethical person has a sense of responsibility toward others and always tries to do what is right. Ethics and laws are extremely important in health care. They protect people receiving care and guide people giving care. Nursing assistants should be guided by a code of ethics. They must know the laws that apply to their jobs.

Examples of legal and ethical behavior by nursing assistants include the following:

- being honest at all times
- protecting residents' privacy
- never becoming personally involved
- reporting abuse or suspected abuse of a resident or assisting a resident in reporting abuse
- never performing unassigned tasks

- reporting all resident observations and incidents
- documenting accurately and on time
- following Standard Precautions (See chapter 2.)

Residents' rights relate to how residents must be treated while living in a facility. They provide an ethical code of conduct for healthcare workers. In 1987 the **OBRA** (Omnibus Budget Reconciliation Act) law was passed by the federal government. It established minimum standards for nursing assistant training. This law identified the following rights:

Quality of life: This means that residents have the right to the best care available. Dignity, choice, and independence are an important part of this.

Services and activities to maintain a high level of wellness: Residents must receive the correct care. Their care should keep them as healthy as possible every day.

Be fully informed regarding rights and services: Residents must be told what care and services are available. They must be aware of all their legal rights.

Participate in their own care: Residents have the right to refuse medication, treatment, and restraints. They also have the right to be informed of changes in their condition.

Make independent choices: Residents can make choices about the care and treatments they receive. They can make personal decisions, such as what to wear and how to spend their time.

Privacy and confidentiality: Residents can expect privacy with care given. Their medical and personal information cannot be discussed with anyone but the healthcare team.

Dignity, respect and freedom: Residents must be respected by caregivers who care for them. Residents cannot be abused in any way.

Security of possessions: Residents' personal possessions must be safe at all times. They cannot be taken or used by persons without a resident's permission.

Choices regarding transfers and discharges: Changes in a resident's location must be done with the resident's knowledge and his or her permission.

Voice complaints: Residents have the right to complain without fear of punishment. Nursing homes must work quickly to try to resolve complaints (Fig. 1-13).

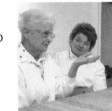

Fig. 1-13. Residents have the right to complain and have their complaints resolved.

Visitations from physician and family: Residents have the right to visits from family, physicians, and other visitors (Fig. 1-14).

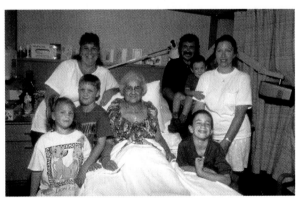

Fig. 1-14. Residents have the right to visitors.

You can help protect your residents' rights in the following ways:

- Watch for and report any signs of abuse or neglect.

- Involve residents in your planning.
- Always explain a procedure before performing it.
- Never abuse a resident physically, emotionally, verbally, or sexually.
- Respect a resident's refusal of care. However, report the refusal to the nurse immediately.
- Tell the nurse if a resident has questions about the goals of care or the care plan.
- Be truthful when documenting care.
- Never talk or gossip about a resident.
- Never enter a resident's room without knocking and asking for permission.
- Never accept gifts or money (Fig. 1-15).

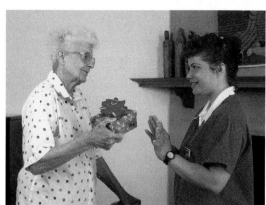

Fig. 1-15. Nursing assistants should not accept money or gifts because it is unprofessional and leads to conflict.

- Never open a resident's mail or look through his belongings.
- Respect residents' personal possessions.
- Report observations regarding a resident's condition or care.
- Assist the resident in resolving any disputes by reporting to your supervisor.

Abuse means purposely causing physical, mental, or emotional pain or injury to someone. Shoving a resident is an example of physical abuse. Purposely embarrassing a resident is an example of emotional or psychological abuse.

Neglect means failing to provide needed care. Deliberately ignoring a resident is an example of neglect.

Domestic violence is abuse by spouses or intimate partners. It can be physical, sexual, or emotional. The victim of the abuse can be a woman, man, elderly person, or a child.

Workplace violence is abuse by an employee or a resident. It can be verbal, physical, or sexual. This includes inappropriate touching and any discussions about sexual subjects.

Negligence means the failure to provide the proper care for a resident that results in unintended injury. Some examples of negligence include

- You do not notice that your resident's dentures do not fit properly. Therefore, he is not eating well. He becomes malnourished.
- You forget to lock a resident's wheelchair before transferring her. She falls and is injured.

If you suspect abuse or neglect, you are legally required to report it.

OBSERVING AND REPORTING
Abuse and Neglect

Physical abuse—the following suspicious injuries should be reported:

- burns
- teeth marks
- bruises on upper arms, lower back, buttocks, and legs
- bone injuries
- scratches and puncture wounds

Signs that could indicate abuse include

- complaints of anxiety
- signs of stress

- withdrawal from others (Fig. 1-16)

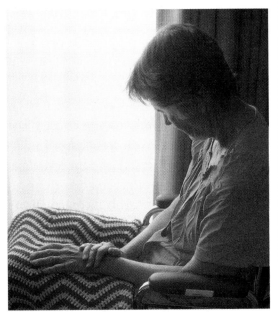

Fig. 1-16. Withdrawing from others is an important change to report.

- fear of family members, friends, or authority figures
- constant pain
- afraid to be alone
- yelling obscenities
- threatening to hurt others
- alcohol or drug abuse

Signs that could indicate neglect include

- pressure sores (See chapter 5 for more information.)
- body not clean
- unanswered call lights
- soiled bedding or briefs not being changed
- weight loss
- poor appetite
- dehydration

If a resident wants to make a complaint of abuse, you must assist in every possible way. This includes informing him or her of the process and his or her rights.

An ombudsman can assist residents too. An **ombudsman** is a legal advocate for residents who visits the facility and listens to residents. He or she decides what course of action to take if there is a problem. Ombudsmen provide an ongoing presence in nursing homes. They monitor care and conditions.

Confidentiality means keeping private things private. As a nursing assistant, you will probably learn a great deal of confidential information about your residents. You may learn about a resident's state of health, finances, and personal and family relationships. You are both ethically and legally obligated keep this information confidential. This means you should not tell anyone other than members of the healthcare team anything about your residents. Your residents have to trust you, and talking about them betrays this trust.

Invasion of privacy is a legal term that means violating someone's right to privacy by exposing his or her private affairs, name, or photograph to the public without that person's consent. Discussing a resident's care or personal affairs with anyone other than your supervisor or another member of the healthcare team could be considered an invasion of privacy, which violates civil law.

Examples:

- A visitor points at a resident in bed and asks you, "What's wrong with him?" You cannot discuss this information with the visitor.

- You are having dinner with your friends at a restaurant. One of them asks, "Anything interesting happen with your residents today?" You are not allowed to discuss this with them.

Any discussion about a resident with team members should be held in a private area, out of hearing distance of other people.

Unit 8: Explain legal aspects of the resident's medical record

The resident's medical record is a legal document. There are legal aspects of your documentation. Careful charting is important for the following reasons:

1. It is the only way to guarantee clear and complete communication between all the members of the care team.

2. Documentation is a legal record of every part of a resident's treatment. Medical charts can be used in court as legal evidence.

3. Documentation protects you and your employer from liability by proving what you did.

4. Documentation on the resident's record provides an up-to-date record of each of your residents' status and care (Fig. 1-16).

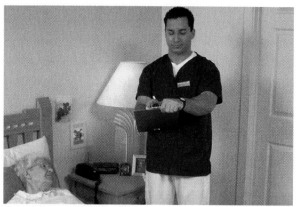

Fig. 1-16. Documentation provides important information about the resident.

GUIDELINES
Careful Documentation

- Write your notes immediately after the care is given. This helps you not to forget important details.

- Think about what you want to say before writing. This will help you be as brief and as clear as possible.

- Write facts, not opinions.

- Write as neatly as you can. Use black ink.

- If you make a mistake, draw one line through it and write the correct word or words. Above the crossed out mistake, write "error" and put your initials and the date. Never erase something you have written. Never use correction fluid (Fig. 1-17).

- Sign your full name and title. Write the correct date.

- Document as specified in the care plan. Some facilities have a "check-off" sheet for documenting care. It is also called an ADL (activities of daily living) sheet.

| 0930 | Changed bed linens, |
| 0945 | VS -BP 190/70 RA error CA BP 150/70 RA |

Connie Acosta, NA
Signature & Title

Fig. 1-17.

TWO

Foundations of Resident Care

Unit 1: Understand the importance of verbal and written communications

Unit 2: Describe barriers to communication

Unit 3: List guidelines for communicating with residents with special needs

Unit 4: Identify ways to promote safety and handle non-medical emergencies

Unit 5: Demonstrate how to recognize and respond to medical emergencies

Unit 6: Describe and demonstrate infection control practices

Unit 1: Understand the importance of verbal and written communications

Effective communication is a critical part of your job. Nursing assistants must communicate with supervisors, members of the healthcare team, residents, and family members. A resident's health depends on how well you communicate your observations and concerns to the nurse.

Communication is the process of exchanging information with others. It includes sending and receiving messages. People communicate using signs and symbols, such as words, drawings, and pictures. They also communicate by their behavior.

Communication can be **verbal**, such as written or spoken messages. Oral reports are an example of verbal communication. Communication can also be nonverbal. In **nonverbal communication**, we do not use words. Examples include shaking your head or shrugging your shoulders. Nonverbal communication changes the message. Be aware of your body language and gestures when you speak (Fig. 2-1). A resident may speak a different language. You may need to use pictures or gestures to communicate.

Nursing assistants must be able to make brief and accurate oral and written presentations to residents and staff. Good communi-

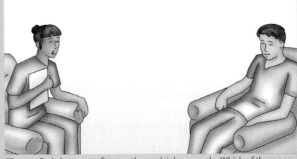

Fig. 2-1. Body language often speaks as plainly as words. Which of these people seems more interested in the conversation they are having?

cation skills are needed to collect information about the resident. Communicating with residents or their family gives you information important to the care team. This information may be written or given in oral reports from one shift to the next. Remember that all resident information you gather is confidential. Only share information with members of the healthcare team.

Reports of a resident's status are used in two ways. The first is to report something the nurse needs to know about immediately. Signs and symptoms that should be reported will be discussed throughout this book. In addition, anything that endangers your resident should be reported immediately. Some examples are:

- falls
- chest pain
- severe headache
- difficulty breathing
- abnormal pulse, respiration, or blood pressure
- change in resident's mental status
- sudden weakness or loss of mobility
- high fever
- loss of consciousness
- change in level of consciousness
- bleeding
- change in resident's condition
- bruises, abrasions, or other signs of possible abuse

When residents report symptoms, events, or feelings, have them repeat what they have said. Ask them for more information. Avoid asking questions that can be answered with a simple "yes" or "no." Instead, ask questions that ask for more detailed information.

For example, asking, "Did you sleep well last night?" could easily be answered "yes" or "no." However, "Tell me about your night and how you slept," will encourage the resident to offer facts and details.

Communicating with Residents

When communicating with your residents, remember these guidelines:

- *Always greet the resident by his or her preferred name.*
- *Identify yourself to the resident.*
- *Focus on the appropriate topic to be discussed.*
- *Face the resident while speaking to him or her. Avoid talking off into space.*
- *Talk with the resident while giving care.*
- *Listen and respond appropriately when the resident speaks.*
- *Praise the resident and smile often.*
- *Encourage the resident to interact with you and others.*
- *Be courteous when communicating.*
- *Always tell the resident when you are leaving the room.*

RЯ *Never refer to a resident by disrespectful terms such as "sweetie" or "honey."*

When making any report, you must collect the right kind of information before documenting it. Facts, not opinions, are most useful to the nurse and the care team. Two kinds of factual information are appropriate in your reporting. **Objective information** is based on what you see, hear, touch, or smell. **Subjective information** is something you cannot or did not observe, but that the resident reported to you. An example of objective information is "The resident lost two pounds." A subjective report of the same resident might be "He says he has no appetite." The nurse and care team need factual information in order to make decisions about care and treatment. Both objective and subjective reports are valuable.

In any report, make sure what you observe and what the resident reports to you are clearly noted. In order to report accurately, observe your residents accurately. To observe accurately, use as many senses as possible to gather information (Fig. 2-2). Some examples follow.

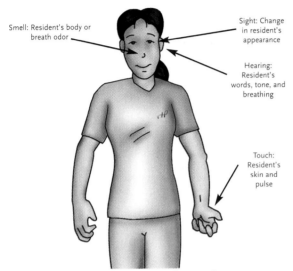

Fig. **2-2.** Reporting what you observe means using more than one sense.

Sight. Look for changes in a resident's appearance. This includes rashes, redness, paleness, swelling, discharge, weakness, sunken eyes, posture or gait (walking) changes.

Hearing. Listen to what the resident tells you about his condition, family, or needs. Is the resident speaking clearly and making sense? Does the resident show emotions, such as anger, frustration, or sadness? Is breathing normal? Does resident wheeze, gasp, or cough? Is the area calm and quiet enough for your resident to rest as needed?

Touch. Does your resident's skin feel hot or cool, moist or dry? Is pulse rate regular?

Smell. Do you notice odor from the resident's body? Odors could suggest inadequate bathing, infections, or incontinence. Incontinence is the inability to control the bladder or bowels. Breath odor could suggest use of alcohol or tobacco, indigestion, or poor oral care.

Using all your senses will allow you to make the most complete report of a resident's situation.

Even for an oral report, you should write notes so you do not forget important details. Following an oral report, document when,

why, about what, and to whom an oral report was given. Use your notes rather than your memory to write these reports.

Sometimes the nurse or another member of the healthcare team will give you a brief oral report on one of your residents. Listen carefully and take notes if you need to (Fig. 2-3). Ask about anything you do not understand. At the end of the conversation, restate what you have been told to make sure you understand it.

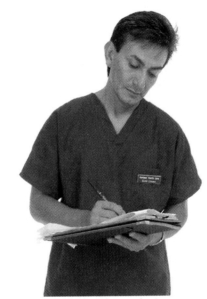

Fig. **2-3.** Take notes on oral reports if you need to.

Throughout your training, you will learn medical terms that describe specific conditions. When communicating with residents and their families, use simple, non-medical terms. But when you communicate with members of the healthcare team, using medical terminology will help you give more complete information. You will find a list of commonly used medical abbreviations in the back of this book.

Unit 2: **Describe barriers to communication**

Communication can be blocked or disrupted in many ways (Fig. 2-4). The following are some barriers and ways to avoid them.

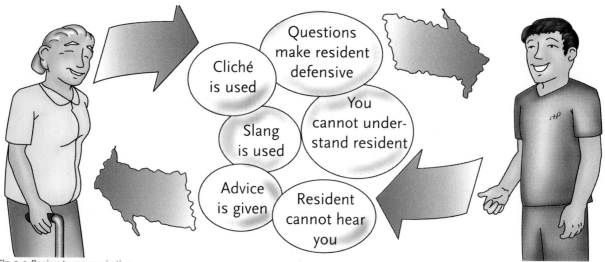

Fig. 2-4. Barriers to communication.

Resident does not hear you, does not hear correctly, or does not understand. Stand directly facing the resident. Speak more slowly than you do with family and friends.

Resident is difficult to understand. Be patient and take time to listen. Ask resident to repeat or explain. Rephrase her message in your own words to make sure you have understood.

Do not use words receiver does not understand. Speak in simple, everyday words. Ask what a word means if you are not sure.

Using slang confuses the message. Avoid using slang words and expressions that may not be understood or are unprofessional.

Avoid clichés. Clichés are phrases that are used over and over again and do not really mean anything.

Giving advice is inappropriate. Do not offer your personal opinion or give advice.

Get to know your residents. Respect what they want to talk about.

Defense mechanisms may be considered barriers to communication. **Defense mech-**

anisms are unconscious behaviors used to release tension or cope with stress. Residents may try to avoid uncomfortable feelings by using a defense mechanism. They include the following:

- Conversion: changing the internal conflict to a physical complaint

- Denial: blocking reality and explaining the situation as a mistake

- Displacement: transferring a strong negative feeling to a safer situation

- Projection: seeing feelings in others that are really our own

- Rationalization: making excuses

Culture can affect communication. Each person's background, values, and language affect how we communicate. When you communicate with residents from different cultures, ask yourself

- What information do I need to communicate to this person?

- Does this person speak English as a first or second language?

- Do I speak this person's language or do I need an interpreter?

- Does this person have any cultural practices about touch or gestures I should adapt to?

Unit 3: **List guidelines for communicating with residents with special needs**

Residents who have special needs require special communication techniques. Special techniques may be required for these conditions or illnesses:

- visual or hearing impairments
- mental illness
- dementia
- combative behavior

Information on communicating with residents who have had a stroke or residents who have dementia, such as Alzheimer's disease, is in chapter 8.

Hearing Impairment

Persons who have impaired hearing or are deaf may have lost their hearing gradually, or they may have been born deaf. Use the following guidelines to make communication more effective.

GUIDELINES
Hearing Impairment

- If the person has a hearing aid, make sure he or she is wearing it and that it is working properly (Fig. 2-5).

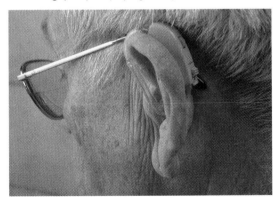

Fig. 2-5. Make sure hearing aids are turned on.

- Reduce or eliminate any background noise, such as televisions, radios, and loud speech. Close doors if you have to.
- Be sure to get the person's attention be-

fore speaking. Do not startle residents by approaching from behind. Walk in front of them or touch them lightly on the arm to let them know you are near.

- Speak clearly, slowly, in good lighting, and while directly facing the person. Do not shout (Fig. 2-6).

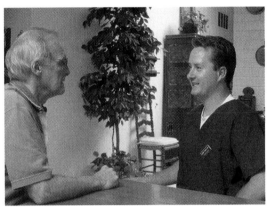

Fig. 2-6. Speak face-to-face in good light.

- Lower the pitch of your voice.
- Know which ear is unaffected and try to speak to that side.
- Use short sentences and simple words.
- Repeat what you have said using different words, when necessary. However, some hearing-impaired persons want you to repeat exactly what was said because they miss only a few words of a sentence.
- Recognize that hearing decline can be a normal aspect of aging. Be matter-of-fact about this. Show your understanding by being supportive.

Vision Impairment

Like hearing impairment, vision impairment can affect people of all ages. It can exist at birth or develop gradually. It can occur in one eye or both. It can also be the result of injury, illness, or aging.

GUIDELINES
Vision Impairment

- If the person has glasses, make sure

they are clean and that he or she wears them. Also, make sure that glasses are in good condition and fit correctly.

ⓖ Identify yourself when you enter the room. Do not touch the resident until you have said your name.

ⓖ Provide adequate lighting at all times.

ⓖ When you enter a new room with the resident, orient him or her to the surroundings.

ⓖ Use the face of an imaginary clock as a guide to explain the position of objects that are in front of resident (Fig. 2-7).

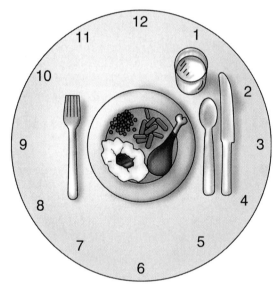

Fig. 2-7. The face of a clock can explain the position of objects.

ⓖ Do not move personal belongings or furniture without the person's knowledge and permission.

ⓖ Offer large-print newspapers, magazines, and books.

ⓖ Encourage the use of the other senses, such as hearing, touch, and smell.

ⓖ Use large clocks, clocks that chime, and radios to help the person keep track of time.

ⓖ Obtain books on tape and any other aids from the local library or support organizations.

Mental Illness

Mental health refers to the normal function of emotional and intellectual abilities. Characteristics of a person who is mentally healthy include the ability to:

• get along with others (Fig. 2-8)

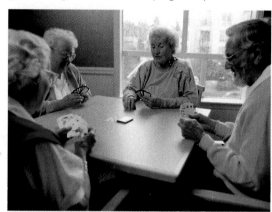

Fig. 2-8. The ability to interact well with other people is a characteristic of mental health.

• adapt to change, care for self and others, and give and accept love

• deal with situations that cause anxiety, disappointment, and frustration

• take responsibility for decisions, feelings, and actions

• control and fulfill desires and impulses appropriately

Although it involves the emotions and mental functions, mental illness is a disease similar to any physical disease. It produces signs and symptoms and affects the body's ability to function. It responds to appropriate treatment and care. Mental illness disrupts a person's ability to function at a normal level in the family, home, or community. It often produces inappropriate behavior. Different types of mental illness can change how well residents communicate.

Mentally healthy people are able to control their emotions and their responses to people and situations. Mentally ill people usually do not have this control. Knowing that mental illness is a disease much like any physical illness helps you work with residents who suffer from mental illness.

GUIDELINES
Mental Illness

- Do not talk to adults as if they were children.

- Use simple, clear statements and a normal tone of voice.

- Be sure that what you say and how you say it shows respect and concern.

- Sit or stand at a normal distance from the resident. Always be aware of your body language.

- Be honest and straightforward, as you would with any resident.

- Avoid arguments.

- Maintain eye contact.

- Listen carefully (Fig. 2-9).

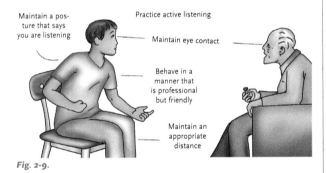

Maintain a posture that says you are listening

Practice active listening

Maintain eye contact

Behave in a manner that is professional but friendly

Maintain an appropriate distance

Fig. 2-9.

Combative Behavior

Residents may sometimes display **combative**, meaning violent or hostile, behavior. Such behavior may include hitting, pushing, kicking, or verbal attacks. Such behavior may be the result of disease affecting the brain. It may also be an expression of frustration. It may just be part of someone's personality. In general, combative behavior is not a reaction to you. Do not take it personally.

Always report combative behavior to your supervisor. Document it. Even if you do not

find the behavior upsetting, the healthcare team needs to be aware of it.

GUIDELINES
Combative Behavior

- Block physical blows or step out of the way, but never hit back (Fig. 2-10).

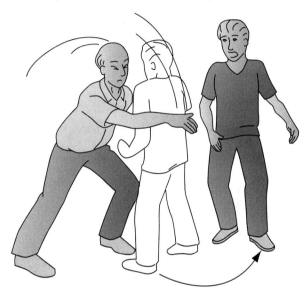

Fig. 2-10. Step out of the way but never hit back.

- Leave the resident alone if you can safely do so.

- Do not respond to verbal attacks.

- Consider what provoked the resident.

- Report inappropriate behavior to the nurse.

Unit 4: **Identify ways to promote safety and handle non-medical emergencies**

Safety

Prevention is the key to safety. Report unsafe conditions to your supervisor *before* accidents occur. As you work, watch for safety hazards. Before leaving a resident's room, look around and do a final check. Ask yourself:

- Is the call light within reach?

- Is the room tidy? Are the resident's items in their proper places?

- Are the side rails up if they are ordered?

- Is the furniture in the same place as you found it? Is the bed in its lowest position?

- Does the resident have a clear walkway around the room and into the bathroom?

📋 *Staff have the responsibility to keep the resident safe from harm. The state agency survey team will look for safety hazards in the environment.*

Principles of Body Mechanics

Body mechanics is the way the parts of the body work together whenever you move. When used properly, good body mechanics can save energy and prevent injury.

The ABC's of good body mechanics are

- **Alignment**. When standing, sitting, or lying down, try to have your body in alignment. This means that the two sides of the body are mirror images of each other. Maintain correct body alignment when lifting or carrying an object by keeping the object close to your body. Point your feet and body in the direction you are moving. Avoid twisting at the waist.

- **Base of support**. The feet are the body's base of support. This means they are the foundation that supports you when you stand. The wider your support, the more stable you are. Standing with legs apart allows for a greater base of support. This person is more stable than someone standing with the feet close together.

- **Center of gravity**. The center of gravity in your body is the point where the most weight is concentrated. This point will depend on the position the body is in. When you stand, your weight is centered in your pelvis. A low center of

gravity also gives a more stable base of support (Fig. 2-11).

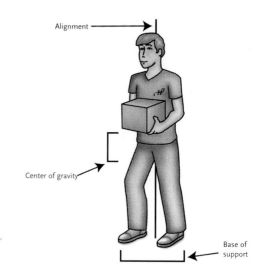

Fig. 2-11. Proper body alignment is important when standing and when sitting.

Common examples of using good body mechanics include the following:

- **Lifting a heavy object from the floor.** Spread your feet shoulder-width apart and bend your knees. Using the strong, large muscles in your thighs, upper arms, and shoulders, lift the object. Pull it close to your body, to a point level with your pelvis. By doing this you are keeping the object close to your center of gravity and base of support. When you stand up, push with your strong hip and thigh muscles to raise your body and the object together (Fig. 2-12).

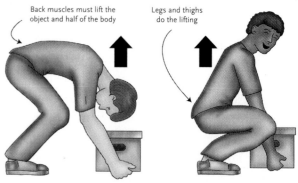

Fig. 2-12. In this illustration, which person is lifting correctly?

- **Do not twist when you are moving an object.** Always face the object or person you are moving. Pivot your feet instead of twisting at the waist.

- **Helping a resident sit up, stand up, or walk**. Whenever you support a resident's weight, protect yourself by assuming a good stance. Place your feet 12 inches, or hip-width apart, one foot in front of the other, and knees bent. Your upper body should stay upright and in alignment.

- **Bend your knees to lower yourself rather than bending from the waist**. Anytime a task requires bending, use a good stance. This uses the big muscles in your legs and hips rather than straining the smaller muscles in your lower back.

- **If you are making a bed, adjust the height to a safe working level, usually waist high**. Avoid bending at the waist.

Keep the following tips in mind to avoid strain and injury:

- Use both arms and hands when lifting, pulling, pushing, or carrying objects.

- Hold objects close to you when you are lifting or carrying them (Fig. 2-13).

- Push, slide, or pull objects rather than lifting them.

- Avoid bending and reaching as much as possible. Move or position furniture so that you do not have to bend or reach.

- When moving a resident, let him know what you will do so he can help if possible. Count to three and lift or move on three so everyone moves together.

- Report to the nurse if your assignments include tasks that you feel you cannot safely perform. Never attempt to lift an object or a resident that you feel you cannot handle.

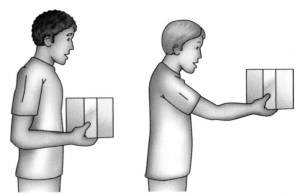

Fig. 2-13. Holding things close to you moves weight toward your center of gravity. In this illustration, whose arms will tire first?

Accident Prevention

Falls

Falls are among the most common accidents. Falls can be caused by an unsafe environment or by loss of abilities. Falls are particularly common among the elderly. Older people are often more seriously injured by falls because their bones are more fragile.

If a resident starts to fall, be in a good position to help support him or her. Never try to catch a falling resident. Rather, use your body to slide him or her to the floor. If you try to reverse a fall, you will probably injure yourself and/or the resident.

Factors that raise the risk of falls include

- clutter
- throw rugs
- exposed electrical cords
- slippery or wet floors
- uneven floors or stairs
- poor lighting
- call lights that are not within reach

Personal conditions that raise the risk of falls include medications, loss of vision, gait or balance problems, weakness, partial paralysis, and disorientation. **Disorientation** means confusion about time or place.

Follow these guidelines to guard against falls:

- Clear all walkways of clutter, throw rugs, and cords.

- Use non-skid mats or carpeting where appropriate. Have resident wear non-skid shoes.

- Keep frequently used personal items close to resident.

- Answer call lights promptly.

- Immediately clean up spills on the floor.

- Mark uneven flooring or stairs with red tape to indicate a hazard.

- Improve lighting where necessary.

- Know residents who are at risk for falls and provide help.

Burns

Burns can be caused by stoves and electrical appliances, hot water or liquids, or heating devices. Small children, older adults, or people with loss of sensation due to paralysis are at greatest risk of burns. Follow these guidelines to guard against burns:

- Always check water temperature with water thermometer or on wrist before using.

- Report frayed electrical cords or unsafe-looking appliances immediately. Do not use these appliances.

- Check temperatures of liquids on your wrist before serving.

Poisoning

Facilities contain many harmful substances that should not be swallowed. These include cleaning products, paints, medicines, toiletries, and glues. Store harmful products away from confused residents or residents with limited vision. Do not leave cleaning products in residents' rooms. Have the number for the Poison Control Center posted by the telephone.

Poisonous chemicals must be kept in locked rooms or cabinets.

Choking

Choking can occur when eating, drinking or swallowing medication. People who are weak, ill, or unconscious may choke on their own saliva. To guard against choking, residents should eat sitting as upright as possible. Elderly residents with swallowing difficulties may have a special diet with liquids thickened to the consistency of honey or syrup. Thickened liquids are easier to swallow.

Fire

Most facilities have a fire safety plan. All workers need to be familiar with it. Fire and disaster drills help you understand your responsibilities in an emergency. Your supervisor will explain your facility's guidelines. Remember to get the residents to safety first. A fast, calm and confident response by the staff saves lives.

Follow these guidelines to guard against fire:

- Never leave smokers unattended. If residents smoke, make sure they are in the designated area for smoking. Check to be sure that cigarettes are extinguished. Empty ashtrays frequently.

- Every facility will have a fire extinguisher (Fig. 2-14). Know how to use them:

    Pull the pin.

    Aim at the base of fire when spraying.

    Squeeze the handle.

    Sweep back and forth at the base of the fire.

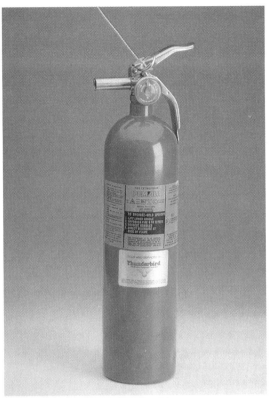

Fig. 2-14. Know how to use a fire extinguisher.

In case of fire, RACE is a good rule to follow:

* **R**emove residents from danger.
* **A**ctivate 911.
* **C**ontain fire if possible.
* **E**xtinguish, or fire department will extinguish.

In addition, follow these guidelines for helping residents exit the building safely:

* Be familiar with the facility's fire evacuation plan.
* Know which residents require one-on-one assistance or assistive devices.
* Remain calm.
* Remove anything blocking a window or door that could be used as a fire exit.
* If clothing catches fire, do not run. Stop, drop to the ground, and roll to extinguish flames.
* Call for emergency help.

Disaster Guidelines

Nursing assistants need to be knowledgeable and responsible during a disaster. An emergency or disaster may occur during working hours. Disasters can include fire, flood, earthquake, hurricane, tornado, or severe weather.

The nurse or administrator will give directions during an emergency. Listen carefully to all directions. Follow instructions. Know the locations of all exits and stairways. Know where the fire alarms and extinguishers are located.

Knowing the appropriate action to take in any situation protects you and your residents. Each facility has a disaster plan developed and available for employees to learn. Make sure you know your facility's plan.

Your instructor will have specific guidelines for disasters that commonly occur in your area.

The facility must have a plan to deal with disasters. The state agency survey team will evaluate staff participation in disaster training and drills.

Unit 5: **Demonstrate how to recognize and respond to medical emergencies**

In this section you will learn how to respond appropriately to medical emergencies. Medical emergencies may be the result of accidents or sudden illnesses. Heart attacks, stroke, diabetic emergencies, choking, automobile accidents, and gunshot wounds are all medical emergencies. Falls, burns, and cuts can also be emergencies when they are severe.

When you come upon an emergency situation, remain calm, act quickly, and communicate clearly. Memorizing the following steps will help you:

- **Assess the situation**. Try to determine what has happened. Make sure you are not in danger. Notice the time.

- **Assess the victim**. Ask the injured or ill person what has happened. If the person is unable to respond, he may be unconscious. To determine whether a person is conscious, tap the person and ask if he is all right. Speak loudly. Use the person's name if you know it. If there is no response, assume the person is unconscious and you have an emergency situation. *Call for help right away, or send someone else to call.*

If a person is conscious and able to speak, then he is breathing and has a pulse. Talk with the person about what happened, and check the person for injury. Check for

- severe bleeding

- changes in consciousness

- irregular breathing

- unusual color or feel to the skin

- swollen places on the body

- anything the resident says is painful

If one of these conditions exists, you may need professional medical help. Always call for help or send someone to get help before doing anything else.

If the injured or ill person is conscious, he may feel panic about his condition. Listen to the person. Tell him what actions are being taken to help him. Be calm and confident to reassure him that he is being taken care of.

Cardiopulmonary resuscitation (CPR) refers to medical procedures used when a person's heart or lungs have stopped working. CPR is used until medical help arrives.

Quick action is necessary. CPR must be started immediately. Brain damage may occur within 4–6 minutes after the heart stops beating and the lungs stop breathing. The person can die within 10 minutes.

Only properly trained people should administer CPR. Your facility should provide you with CPR training. If your facility does not schedule you for training, ask about Heart Association or Red Cross CPR training. CPR is an important skill to learn. If you are not trained, **never** attempt to perform CPR. This textbook is not a CPR course. The following is intended as a brief review for people who have had CPR training:

1. Call for help. Remain calm.

2. Ask the person if he or she is okay.

3. If there is no response, check for breathing.

    - Look for the chest to rise and fall.

    - Listen for sounds of breathing. Put your ear near the person's nose and mouth.

    - Feel for the person's breath on your cheek.

4. Tilt the head back slightly by lifting the lower jaw to open the airway (head tilt-chin lift method) (Fig. 2-15).

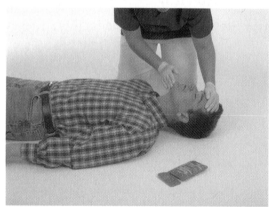

Fig. 2-15.

5. Check for any obstruction to the airway. Clear the airway if there is any blockage.

6. If the person is still not breathing, you will have to breathe for the person. Give two rescue breaths.

7. Pinch the nose to keep air from escaping from the nostrils. Cover the person's mouth completely with your mouth.

8. Blow into the person's mouth, watching for the chest to rise (Fig. 2-16). Blow two full breaths. Turn your head to the side to listen for air.

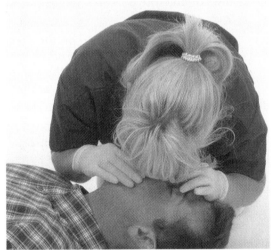

Fig. 2-16.

9. Check for pulse by gently feeling the carotid artery in the neck for 5–10 seconds (Fig. 2-17). If there is no pulse, give 15 chest compressions only if you have been trained to do so. Be sure the person is lying flat on a hard surface.

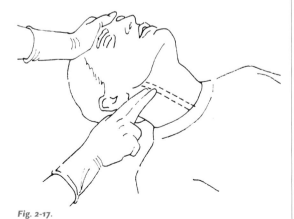

Fig. 2-17.

- Find the lower end of the person's sternum. Do this by following the rib cage up to the center of the chest.

- Place your index finger next to your middle finger where the ribs meet the sternum. Place the heel of your other hand next to the upper finger over the lower half of the sternum (Fig. 2-18).

- Place the heel of your hand on top of the positioned hand. Interlace your fingers.

- Use the heels of your hands to give 15 chest compressions.

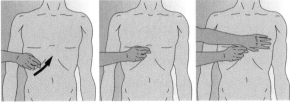

Fig. 2-18.

10. Continue giving two breaths followed by 15 compressions until medical help arrives.

When medical help arrives follow their directions. Assist them as necessary.

When something is blocking the tube through which air enters the lungs, the person has an **obstructed airway** . When people are choking, they usually put their hands to their throats and cough (Fig. 2-19). As long as the person can speak, breathe, or cough, do nothing. Encourage him to cough as forcefully as possible to get the object out. Stay with the person at all times, until he stops choking or can no longer speak, breathe, or cough.

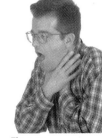

Fig. 2-19.

If a person can no longer speak, breathe, or cough, call for help immediately. After calling for help return to the person.

The Heimlich maneuver is a procedure used for choking. It uses abdominal thrusts to remove the blockage upward, out of the throat. Make sure the person needs help before starting the Heimlich maneuver. If the person cannot speak or cough, or if his response is weak, start the Heimlich maneuver.

Heimlich Maneuver for the Conscious Person

1. Stand behind the person and bring your arms under his arms. Wrap your arms around the person's waist.

2. Make a fist with one hand. Place the flat, thumb side of the fist against the person's abdomen, above the navel but below the breastbone.

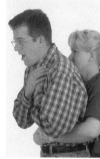

3. Grasp the fist with your other hand. Pull both hands toward you and up, quickly and forcefully (Fig. 2-20).

Fig. 2-20.

4. Repeat until the object is pushed out or the person loses consciousness.

If the person becomes unconscious while choking, help him to the floor gently, lying on his back with his face up. Make sure help is on its way. He probably has a completely blocked airway and needs professional medical help immediately.

Heimlich Maneuver for the Unconscious Person

1. Make sure the person is on his back.

2. Open the airway by tilting the head back and lifting the chin.

3. Check for breath.

4. If there is no breathing, open the mouth and try to sweep the mouth with your finger to remove the blockage. Sweep along the inside of the mouth toward the base of the tongue (Fig. 2-21).

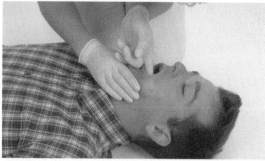

Fig. 2-21.

5. Pinch the nose closed and give two full breaths.

6. If air still does not enter the airway, kneel and straddle the person's thighs, facing his face.

7. Place the heel of one hand on the person's abdomen, slightly above the navel, with your fingers pointing toward the person's chest. Place your other hand over the first hand.

8. Give five abdominal thrusts by pushing your hands inward and upward (Fig. 2-22).

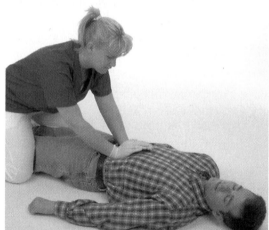

Fig. 2-22.

9. Check to see if the blockage is removed.

10. Try to sweep the object out with your fingers.

11. Repeat steps 5–9 if necessary.

Shock

Shock occurs when organs and tissues in the body do not receive an adequate blood supply. Bleeding, heart attack, severe infection, and conditions that cause the blood pressure to fall can lead to shock. Shock can become worse when the person is extremely frightened or in severe pain.

Shock is a dangerous, life-threatening situation. Signs of shock include pale or bluish skin, staring, increased pulse and respiration rates, decreased blood pressure, and extreme thirst. Always call for help if you suspect a person is experiencing shock. To prevent or treat shock, do the following.

Shock

1. Have the person lie down on her back. If the person is bleeding from the mouth or vomiting, place her on her side (unless you suspect that the neck, back, or spinal cord is injured).

2. Control bleeding. This procedure is described later in the chapter.

3. Check pulse and respirations if possible. (See chapter 6.)

4. Keep the person as calm and comfortable as possible.

5. Maintain normal body temperature. If the weather is cold, place a blanket around the person. If the weather is hot, provide shade.

6. Elevate the feet unless the person has a head or abdominal injury, breathing difficulties, or a fractured bone or back (Fig. 2-23). Elevate the head and shoulders if a head wound or breathing difficulties are present. Never elevate a body part if a broken bone exists.

7. Do not give the person anything to eat or drink.

8. Call for help immediately. Victims of shock should always receive medical care as soon as possible.

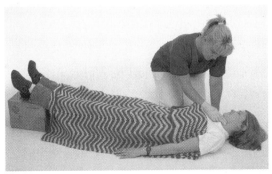

Fig. 2-23.

Insulin Shock and Diabetic Coma

Insulin shock and diabetic coma are complications of diabetes that can be life-threatening. Insulin shock can result from either too much insulin or too little food. It occurs when a dose of insulin is administered and the person skips a meal or does not eat all the food required. Even when a regular amount of food is eaten, physical activity may rapidly metabolize the food so that too much insulin is in the body. Vomiting and diarrhea may also lead to insulin shock in people with diabetes.

The first signs of insulin shock include feeling weak or different, nervousness, dizziness, and perspiration. See list below for further signs. These signal that the resident needs food in a form that can be rapidly absorbed. Call the nurse if the resident has shown signs of insulin shock.

The following are signs and symptoms of insulin shock:

- hunger
- weakness
- rapid pulse
- headache
- low blood pressure
- perspiration
- cold, clammy skin
- confusion
- trembling
- nervousness
- blurred vision
- numbness of the lips and tongue
- unconsciousness

Having too little insulin causes diabetic coma. It can result from undiagnosed diabetes, going without insulin or not taking

Foundations of Resident Care

enough, eating too much food, not getting enough exercise, and physical or emotional stress.

The signs of onset of diabetic coma include increased thirst or urination, abdominal pain, deep or labored breathing, and breath that smells sweet or fruity. Call the nurse immediately if you think your resident is experiencing diabetic coma.

Other signs and symptoms of diabetic coma include the following:

- hunger
- weakness
- rapid, weak pulse
- headache
- low blood pressure
- dry skin
- flushed cheeks
- drowsiness
- slow, deep, and labored breathing
- nausea and vomiting
- abdominal pain
- sweet, fruity breath odor
- air hunger, or resident gasping for air and being unable to catch his breath
- unconsciousness

See chapter 8 for more information on diabetes and related care.

CVA or Stroke

A cerebrovascular accident (CVA), or stroke, is caused when a clot or a ruptured blood vessel suddenly cuts off blood supply to the brain. Symptoms that a stroke is beginning may include dizziness, ringing in the ears, blurred vision, headache, nausea, vomiting, slurring of words, and loss of memory. These signs and symptoms should be reported immediately.

A transient ischemic attack, or TIA, is a warning sign of a CVA. It is the result of a temporary lack of oxygen in the brain and may last several days, weeks, or months. Symptoms include tingling, weakness, or some loss of movement in an arm or leg. These symptoms should not be ignored. Report any of these symptoms to the nurse immediately.

Signs that a stroke is occurring include any of the following:

- loss of consciousness
- redness in the face
- noisy breathing
- dizziness
- blurred vision
- ringing in the ears
- headache
- nausea/vomiting
- seizures
- loss of bowel and bladder control
- paralysis on one side of the body
- weakness on one side of the body
- the inability to speak or to speak clearly
- use of inappropriate words
- elevated blood pressure
- slow pulse rate

See chapter 8 for more information on strokes.

Myocardial Infarction or Heart Attack

When blood flow to the heart is completely blocked, oxygen and nutrients fail to reach its cells. Waste products are not removed and the muscle cell dies. This is called a myocardial infarction (MI), or heart attack. The area of dead tissue may be large or small, depending on the artery involved.

A myocardial infarction is an emergency that can result in serious heart damage or death. The following are signs and symptoms of MI:

- sudden, severe pain in the chest, usually on the left side or in the center, behind the sternum

- a feeling of indigestion or heartburn

- nausea and vomiting

- dyspnea, or difficulty breathing

- dizziness

- discoloration of the skin; it may be pale, gray, or blue

- perspiration

- cold and clammy skin

- weak and irregular pulse rate

- low blood pressure

- anxiety and a sense of impending doom

The pain of a heart attack is commonly described as a crushing, pressing, squeezing, stabbing, piercing pain, or "like someone is sitting on my chest." The pain may go down the inside of the left arm. A person may also feel it in the neck and/or in the jaw. The pain does not go away.

You must take immediate action if a resident experiences any of these symptoms. Follow these steps.

Heart Attack

1. Call or have someone call the nurse.

2. Place the person in a comfortable position. Encourage him to rest, and reassure him that you will not leave him alone.

3. Loosen clothing around the neck (Fig. 2-24).

4. Do not give the person liquids.

5. If the person takes heart medication, such as nitroglycerin, find the medication and

offer it to him. **Never place medication in someone's mouth.**

6. Monitor the person's breathing and pulse. If the person stops breathing or has no pulse, perform rescue breathing or CPR if you are trained to do so.

7. Stay with the person until help arrives.

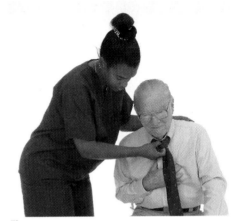

Fig. 2-24.

Fainting

Fainting occurs when the blood supply drops, causing a loss of consciousness. Fainting may be the result of hunger, fear, pain, fatigue, standing for a long time, poor ventilation, or overheating.

Signs and symptoms of fainting include dizziness, perspiration, pale skin, weak pulse, shallow respirations, and blackness in the visual field. If someone appears likely to faint, follow these steps.

Fainting

1. Have the person lie down or sit down before fainting occurs.

2. If the person is in a sitting position, have him bend forward and place his head between his knees (Fig. 2-25). If the person is lying flat on his back, elevate the legs.

3. Report the incident to the nurse.

4. Loosen any tight clothing.

5. Have the person stay in position for at least five minutes after symptoms disappear.

6. Help the person get up slowly. Continue to observe him for symptoms of fainting.

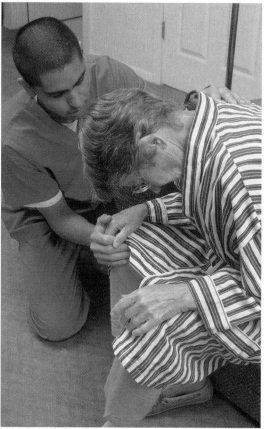

Fig. 2-25.

During a seizure, a person may shake severely and thrust arms and legs uncontrollably (Fig. 2-26). He may clench his jaw, drool, and be unable to swallow. The following emergency measures should be taken if a resident has a seizure.

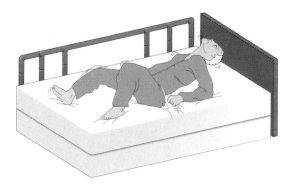

Fig. 2-26.

Seizures

1. Lower the person to the floor.
2. Have someone call the nurse immediately. Do not leave the person during the seizure unless you must do so to get medical help.
3. Move furniture away to prevent injury. If a pillow is nearby, place it under his or her head.
4. Do not try to restrain the person.
5. Do not force anything between the person's teeth. Do not place your hands in the person's mouth for any reason. You could be bitten.
6. Do not give liquids.
7. When the seizure is over, check breathing.
8. Report the length of the seizure and your observations to the nurse.

If a person does faint, lower him to the floor or other flat surface. Position him on his back. Elevate his legs 8 to 12 inches. Loosen any tight clothing. Check to make sure the person is breathing. He should recover quickly, but keep him lying down for several minutes. Report the incident to the nurse immediately. Fainting may be a sign of a more serious medical condition.

Seizures

Seizures are involuntary, often violent, contractions of muscles. They can involve a small area or the entire body. Seizures are caused by an abnormality in the brain. They can occur in young children who have a high fever. Older children and adults who have a serious illness, fever, head injury, or epilepsy may also have seizures.

The main goal of a caregiver during a seizure is to make sure the resident is safe.

Bleeding

Severe bleeding can cause death quickly and must be controlled. Call the nurse immediately, then follow these steps to control bleeding.

Bleeding

1. Put on gloves.
2. Hold a thick sterile pad, a clean pad, or a clean cloth such as a handkerchief or towel against the wound. Have the injured person

use his bare hand until you can get a clean pad. Also have the resident hold the pad if he is able until you can put on gloves.

3. Press down hard directly on the bleeding wound until help arrives. Do not decrease pressure (Fig. 2-27). Put additional pads over the first pad if blood seeps through. Do not remove the first pad.

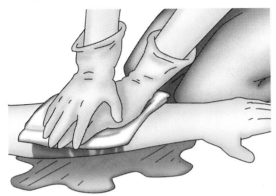

Fig. 2-27

4. Raise the wound above the heart to slow down the bleeding. If the wound is on an arm, leg, hand, or foot, and there are no broken bones, prop up the limb on towels, blankets, coats, or other absorbent material.

5. When bleeding is under control, secure the dressing to keep it in place. Check the person for symptoms of shock (pale skin, increased pulse and respiration rates, decreased blood pressure, and extreme thirst). Stay with the person until help arrives.

6. Wash hands thoroughly when finished.

Once a medical emergency is over, you will have to file an incident/accident report with your facility. Report according to your facility's guidelines. It is helpful to know in advance what information you will need complete the report.

Unit 6: **Describe and demonstrate infection control practices**

Asepsis means no infection is present. It refers to the clean conditions you want to create in your facility. Preventing the spread of infection is important. Know your facility's specific infection control practices. They are

in place to protect you, your residents, and others from disease.

Infections occur when harmful microorganisms, called **pathogens**, enter the body. To understand how to prevent disease you must first understand how it is spread.

The **chain of infection** is a way of describing how disease is transmitted from one living being to another (Fig. 2-28). Definitions and examples of each of the six links in the chain of infection follow.

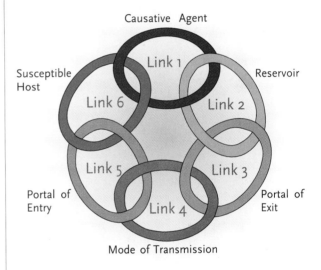

Fig. 2-28. The chain of infection.

Link 1: **Causative agent** (pathogen or microorganism that causes disease): bacteria, viruses, fungi, protozoa

Link 2: **Reservoir** (place where the pathogen lives and grows): the lungs, blood, large intestine, etc.

Link 3: **Portal of exit** (any body opening on infected person that allows pathogens to leave): nose, mouth, eyes, cut in skin (Fig. 2-29)

Link 4: **Mode of transmission** (how the pathogen travels from one person to the next): through the air, getting on body (direct contact) or other surfaces (indirect contact)

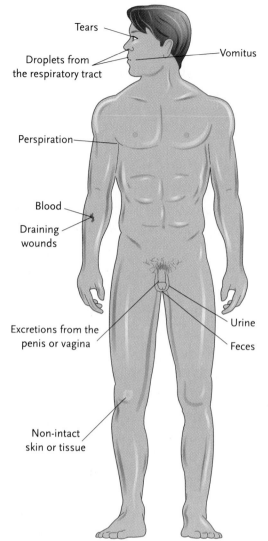

Fig. 2-29. Portals of exit.

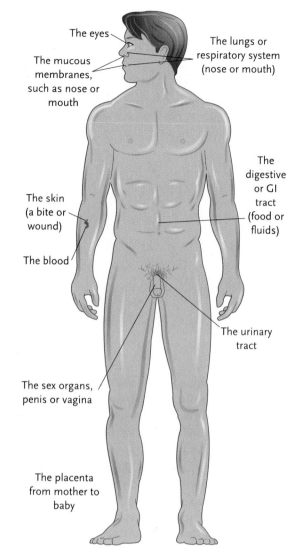

Fig. 2-30. Portals of entry.

Link 5: **Portal of entry** (any body opening on uninfected person that allows pathogens to enter): nose, mouth, eyes, other mucous membranes, cut in skin, or dry/cracked skin (Fig. 2-30)

Link 6: **Susceptible host** (uninfected person who could get sick): all healthcare workers and anyone in their care who is not already infected with that particular disease

If one of the links in the chain of infection is broken, then the spread of infection is stopped. By using infection control practices, you can help stop the pathogens from traveling (Link 4), and getting on your hands,

nose, eyes, mouth, skin, etc. (Link 5). You can also reduce your own chances of getting sick by having immunizations (Link 6) for diseases such as Hepatitis-B and influenza.

Standard Precautions and Transmission-Based Precautions

State and federal government agencies have guidelines and laws concerning infection control. The **Occupational Safety and Health Administration (OSHA)** is a federal government agency that makes rules to protect workers from hazards on the job. The Center for Disease Control issues guidelines for healthcare workers to follow on the job.

In 1996, the Centers for Disease Control (CDC) recommended a comprehensive new infection control system for reducing the risk of contracting infectious diseases. There are two tiers of precautions within this system: Standard Precautions and Transmission-Based Precautions.

Standard Precautions and Transmission-Based Precautions provide a way to stop the spread of infection by interrupting the mode of transmission. In other words, these guidelines do not stop an infected person from giving off pathogens (germs). However, by following these guidelines you help prevent those pathogens from infecting you or other persons in your care.

1. Standard Precautions should ALWAYS be practiced with every single person in your care.

2. Transmission-Based Precautions vary based on how a particular infection is transmitted. These precautions are IN ADDITION to the Standard Precautions. You will learn about these precautions in greater detail later.

Standard Precautions

Standard Precautions include the following measures:

- Wear gloves if you may come into contact with blood, any body fluids or secretions, broken skin (including abrasions, acne, cuts, sutures or stitches, and pinpricks), or mucous membranes (such as the linings of the mouth, nose, eyes, vagina, rectum, and penis). Such situations may include mouth care, bathroom assistance, perineal care, assistance with a bedpan or urinal, cleaning up spills, cleansing urinals, bedpans, and other containers that have held body fluids, and disposing of wastes.

- Remove gloves immediately when finished with procedure.

- Wash your hands before putting on gloves. Wash your hands immediately after removing gloves. Be careful not to touch clean objects with your gloves.

- Immediately wash all skin surfaces that have been contaminated with blood and body fluids.

- Wear a disposable gown if you may come into contact with blood or body fluids.

- Wear a mask and protective glasses if the possibility exists that you will come into contact with splashing blood or body fluids.

- Wear gloves and use caution when handling razor blades, needles, and other sharps.

- Avoid cuts when shaving residents.

- Carefully bag all contaminated supplies. Dispose of them according to your facility's policy.

- Body fluids that are being saved for a specimen should be clearly labeled with the resident's name and a biohazard label. They should be kept in a container with a lid.

- Never attempt to put a cap on a needle or sharp. Dispose of it in an approved container.

- Contaminated wastes should be disposed of according to your facility's policy.

The following body substances and fluids are covered under Standard Precautions:

- Blood and blood products

- All body fluids, secretions, excretions (except sweat)

- Broken skin (including acne and open sores)

Foundations of Resident Care

- Mucous membranes (lining of mouth, nose, eyes, rectum, vagina)

Standard Precautions should ALWAYS be practiced on persons in your care regardless of their infection status. Remember, you cannot tell by how someone looks or acts, or even by reading their chart, whether they carry a bloodborne disease. If you practice Standard Precautions you will significantly reduce the risk of getting any diseases from those persons in your care. You will also keep one resident's infection from harming another resident.

Washing your hands is the single most important thing you can do to prevent the spread of disease to yourself and others! Use lotion to prevent dry, cracked, or irritated skin. If you wear rings, consider removing them during working hours. Rings attract bacteria which becomes difficult to wash off.

Wash hands

- before and after using the restroom
- after touching any body substance
- after handling contaminated items
- before putting on gloves
- immediately after removing gloves
- before feeding residents
- before you eat
- between all contacts with persons in your care
- before leaving the facility

Washing hands

Equipment: soap, paper towels

1. **Turn on water at sink.**

2. **Angle arms down holding hands lower than elbows. Wet hands and wrists thoroughly (Fig. 2-31).**
    The hands are more likely to be contaminated. Water should run from cleanest to dirtiest.

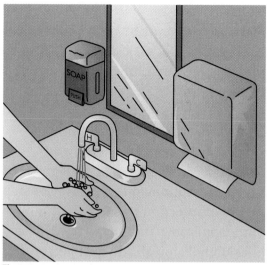

Fig. 2-31.

3. **Apply skin cleanser or soap to hands.**

4. **Lather all surfaces of fingers and hands, including above the wrists, producing friction, for at least 10 seconds (Fig. 2-32).**
    Lather and friction loosen skin oils and allow pathogens to be rinsed away.

5. **Clean nails by rubbing them in palm of other hand.**
    Most pathogens on hands come from beneath the nails.

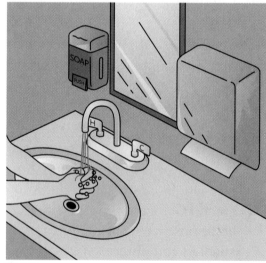

Fig. 2-32.

6. **Rinse all surfaces of hands and wrists, running water down from wrists to fingertips.**
    Wrists are cleanest, fingertips dirtiest. Soap left on skin may cause irritation and rashes.

7. **Use clean, dry paper towel to dry all surfaces of hands, wrists, and fingers.**

8. **Use clean, dry paper towel or clean, dry area of paper towel to turn off faucet, without contaminating hands (Fig. 2-33).**

Hands will be recontaminated if you touch the dirty faucet with clean hands.

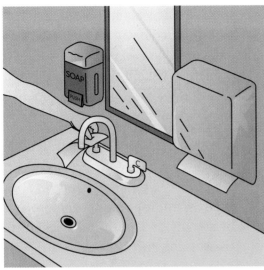

Fig. 2-33.

9. Dispose of used paper towel(s) in wastebasket immediately after shutting off faucet.

☀ *When washing your hands, you must use friction for at least 10 seconds.*

Personal Protective Equipment

Wear gloves

- when touching blood or any body substances

- when performing or assisting with mouth care or care of any mucous membrane

- when performing or assisting with care of the **perineal area** (the area between the genitals and anus)

- when shaving a resident

- when touching broken skin

- when you have open sores or cuts on your hands

- when disposing of soiled bed linens, gowns, dressings, and pads

Change gloves

- immediately before contact with mucous membranes or broken skin

- if gloves become soiled

- if gloves become worn or damaged

Remove gloves

- promptly after use and wash your hands

- before touching non-contaminated items or environmental surfaces

- before caring for another resident

Clean, non-sterile gloves are generally adequate. They may be vinyl or latex. Some people develop allergies to latex. If you do, let the nurse know. Alternative gloves will be provided. Always let the nurse know if you have dry, cracked, or broken skin. Remember to wash hands before and after wearing gloves!

Putting on gloves

1. Wash hands.

2. If right-handed, slide one glove on left hand (reverse, if left-handed).

3. With gloved hand take second glove and slide other hand into the glove.

4. Interlace fingers to smooth out folds and create a comfortable fit.

5. Carefully look for tears, holes, or spots. Replace the glove if necessary.

6. If wearing a gown, pull the cuff of the gloves over the sleeve of gown (Fig. 2-34).

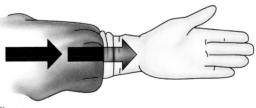

Fig. 2-34.

Remember, you are wearing gloves to protect your skin from becoming contaminated. After giving care, your gloves are contaminated. If you open a door with the gloved hand, the doorknob becomes contaminated.

Later, when you open the door with an ungloved hand, you will be infected even though you wore gloves during the procedure. It is a common mistake to contaminate the room around you. Do not do it. Before touching surfaces such as doorknob, remove gloves. Wash your hands. Afterward, put on new gloves if necessary.

Taking off gloves

1. Touching only the outside of one glove, pull the first glove off by pulling down from the cuff (Fig. 2-35).

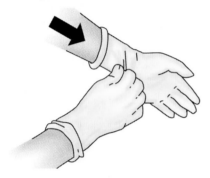

Fig. 2-35.

2. As the glove comes off hand it should be turned inside out.

3. With the fingertips of gloved hand hold the glove that was just removed. With ungloved hand, reach two fingers *inside* the remaining glove. Be careful not to touch any part of the outside (Fig. 2-36).

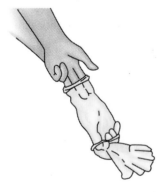

Fig. 2-36.

4. Pull down, turning this glove inside out and over the first glove as it is removed.

5. You should be holding one glove from its clean inner side and the other glove should be inside it.

6. Drop both gloves into the proper container.

7. Wash hands.

In addition to gloves, personal protective equipment (PPE) includes gowns, masks, eye shields (goggles), and face shields. Your facility will provide you with PPE as necessary. However, it is your responsibility to know where it is kept and how to use it.

Wear gowns and aprons

- during a procedure or resident care activity that is likely to cause body fluid splashes or sprays

- that are appropriate for the procedure or activity and amount of body fluid likely to be encountered

Remove the gown as soon as possible and wash your hands.

Clean, non-sterile gowns are adequate to

- protect your exposed skin

- prevent soiling of your clothing

Putting on a gown

1. Wash hands.

2. Open gown. Hold out in front of you and allow gown to open. Do not shake it. Slip your arms into the sleeves and pull gown on (Fig. 2-37).

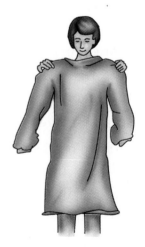

Fig. 2-37.

3. Tie the neck ties into a bow so they can be easily untied later.

4. Reaching behind, pull gown until it com-

pletely covers clothing. Tie the back ties (Fig. 2-38).

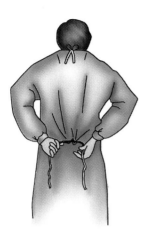

Fig. 2-38.

5.   Remember, use gowns only once and then discard or remove. When removing a gown, roll it dirty side in and away from the body. If gown ever becomes wet or soiled, remove it. Check clothing, and put on a new gown.

6.   Put on gloves after putting on gown.

👁 Some examiners will ask why a gown must be non-permeable. The answer is that if the clothes under the gown become wet, they are considered contaminated.

Wear mask, eye protection, and face shields

•   to protect facial mucous membranes during procedures and resident care activities that are likely to generate splashes or sprays

Putting on a mask and eye shield

1.   Wash hands.

2.   Pick up mask by top strings or elastic strap. Do not touch mask where it touches your face.

3.   Adjust mask over nose and mouth. Tie top strings first, then bottom string. Masks must always be dry or they must be replaced. Never wear a mask hanging from only the bottom tie (Fig. 2-39).

4.   Put on eye shield.

5.   Put on gloves *after* putting on mask and eye shield.

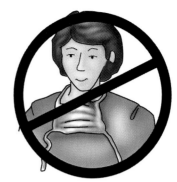

Fig. 2-39.

Change mask between residents.

When applying PPE, remember this order:

1. Apply mask and eye shield.

2. Apply gown.

3. Apply gloves last.

When removing PPE, remember this order:

1. Remove gloves.

2. Remove gown.

3. Remove mask and eye shield.

Equipment and Linen Handling

In health care, an object can only be called "clean" if it has not been contaminated by pathogens. An object that is "dirty" has been contaminated by pathogens. Facilities will have separate areas for clean and dirty items, such as equipment, linen, and supplies. Know the location of these areas and what supplies are stored in each.

Handle all equipment in a manner that prevents:

•   skin/mucous membrane contact

•   contamination of your clothing with the equipment

•   transfer of disease to other residents or environments from the equipment

Do not use "re-usable" equipment again

Foundations of Resident Care

until it has been properly cleaned and re-processed. Dispose of all "single-use" equipment properly.

Clean and disinfect

- all environmental surfaces
- beds, bedrails, all bedside equipment (Fig. 2-40)
- all frequently touched surfaces (such as door knobs)

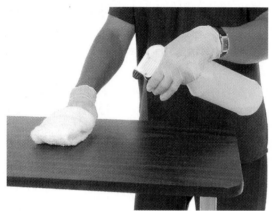

Fig. 2-40.

Handle, transport, and process soiled linens in a manner that prevents

- skin and mucous membrane exposure
- contamination of clothing (hold linen away from uniform) (Fig. 2-41)
- transfer of disease to other residents and environments

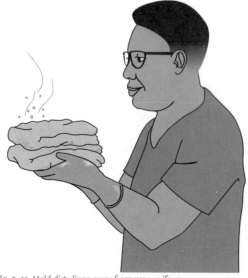

Fig. 2-41. Hold dirty linen away from your uniform.

Transmission-Based Precautions

These are special precautions which should be used for persons in your care who are infected or suspected of being infected with a disease that requires ADDITIONAL precautions beyond the Standard Precautions.

There are three categories of Transmission-Based Precautions are

- Airborne Precautions
- Droplet Precautions
- Contact Precautions

The category that is used depends upon the pathogen that is being isolated.

Three important points to remember are

1. Transmission-Based Precautions are always used IN ADDITION to Standard Precautions.
2. The resident must be reassured that it is the disease, not the person with the disease, that is being isolated. Communicate with your resident. Explain why these special steps are being taken.
3. Facility policies about how to properly discard garbage and soiled linen to remove it from the isolation area must be followed.

Airborne precautions are used for diseases that can be transmitted through the air after being expelled by the resident (Fig. 2-42). The microorganisms are so small that they can attach to moisture in the air and remain floating for some time. For certain care you may be required to wear special masks, such as N95 or HEPA masks, to avoid being infected. Airborne diseases include tuberculosis, measles, and chicken pox.

Droplet precautions are used when the disease-causing microorganism does not stay

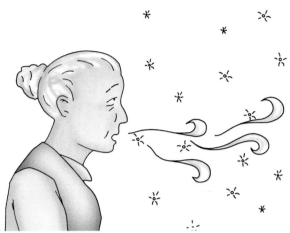

Fig. 2-42. Airborne diseases stay suspended in the air.

suspended in the air and usually travels only short distances after being expelled. Droplets can be generated by coughing, sneezing, talking, laughing, or suctioning (Fig. 2-43).

Droplet precautions can include wearing a face mask during care procedures and restricting visits from uninfected people. Residents should wear masks when being moved from room. Cover your nose and mouth with a tissue when you sneeze or cough and ask residents, family, and others to do the same. If you sneeze on your hands, wash them promptly.

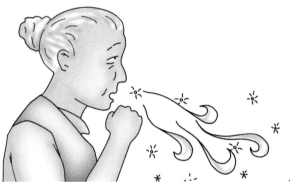

Fig. 2-43. Droplet precautions are followed when the disease causing microorganism does not stay suspended in the air.

Contact precautions are used when the resident is at risk of transmitting or contracting a microorganism from touching an infected object or person (Fig. 2-44). Examples include bacteria that could infect an open skin wound or infection. Lice, scabies (a skin disease that causes itching), and conjunctivitis (pink eye) are other examples. Transmission

can occur with skin-to-skin contact during transfers or bathing. Precautions include PPE and resident isolation. Contact precautions require washing hands with antimicrobial soap, and not touching infected surfaces with ungloved hands or uninfected surfaces with contaminated gloves.

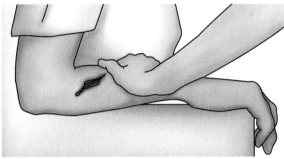

Fig. 2-44. Contact precautions are followed when the person is at risk of transmitting or getting a microorganism from touching an infected object or person.

Spills

Spills can pose a serious risk of infection. Nursing homes will have specific cleaning solutions for spills.

GUIDELINES
Cleaning Spills Involving Blood, Body Fluids, or Glass

- Apply gloves before starting to clean up the spill. In some cases, industrial-strength gloves are best because they will not tear if you are also handling glass.

- Clean up spills immediately with the proper cleaning solution.

- Do not pick up any pieces of broken glass, no matter how large, with your hands. Use a dustpan and broom or other tools.

- Waste containing broken glass, blood, or body fluids should be properly bagged. Put the waste in one trash bag and close it. Then put the first bag inside a second, clean trash bag and close it. Waste containing blood or body fluids may need to be placed in a special biohazard container. Follow your facility's policy.

Foundations of Resident Care

Common Infectious Diseases

The most serious infections include:

- **Tuberculosis (TB)**: TB is a bacterial infection that affects the lungs. It is transmitted through the air. It causes coughing, difficulty breathing, fever, and fatigue. It can be cured. However, if left untreated, it can cause death.

- **Hepatitis** is the inflammation of the liver caused by different viruses. The most common are hepatitis A, B, and C. Hepatitis B and C are bloodborne diseases that can cause death. There is a vaccine for hepatitis B. Your employer will offer you this free vaccine.

- **Methicillin-Resistant Staphylococcus Aureus (MRSA)** is caused by bacteria that are resistant to many antibiotics. MRSA can develop when people do not take all of the medication prescribed to them. MRSA is spread by direct contact with an infected person or indirect contact with contaminated equipment or supplies.

- **Vancomycin-Resistant Enteroccus (VRE)** is also resistance caused by a person not taking all of a powerful antibiotic called Vancomycin.

See chapter 8 for information on Acquired Immunodeficiency Syndrome (AIDS).

Employer-Employee Responsibilities

Employers' responsibilities for infection control include the following:

- Establish infection control procedures and an exposure control plan to protect workers.

- Provide continuing in-service education on infection control, including bloodborne and airborne pathogens.

- Have written procedures to follow should an exposure occur, including medical treatment and plans to prevent similar exposures.

- Provide PPE for employees to use and train them when and how to properly use it.

- Provide free hepatitis B vaccinations for all employees.

Employees' responsibilities for infection control include the following:

- Follow standard precautions.

- Follow all of the facility's policies and procedures.

- Follow care plans and assignments.

- Use provided PPE as indicated or as appropriate.

- Take advantage of the free hepatitis B vaccination.

- Immediately report any exposure you have to infection.

- Participate in annual education programs covering the control of infection.

Staff have the responsibility to prevent the spread of infection. The state agency survey team will look for evidence of staff handwashing and the availability and use of personal protective equipment.

THREE

Understanding Your Residents

Unit 1: Explain why promoting independence and self-care is important

Any big change in lifestyle, such as moving into a nursing home, is emotional. Residents experience fear, loss, and uncertainty with their decline in health and independence. These feelings may cause residents to behave differently than at any other time in their lives. Be aware that dramatic changes in a resident's life may cause anger, hostility, or depression. Be supportive and encouraging. Be patient, understanding, and empathic. **Empathy** is the ability to share an experience and feelings with another by putting yourself in his or her shoes.

To best understand your resident, realize that his or her loss of independence is very difficult. Somebody else must now do what the resident did for himself all of his life. It is also a difficult adjustment for friends and family members. For example, the resident may have been the main provider for his or her family. Or the resident may have been the person who did all of the cooking for the family.

Residents may be experiencing some of the following losses:

- loss of spouse, family members, or friends due to death

- loss of workplace and its relationships due to retirement

- loss of ability to go to places such as lodges, favorite restaurants, clubs, etc.

- loss of familiar home environment and personal possessions (Fig. 3-1)

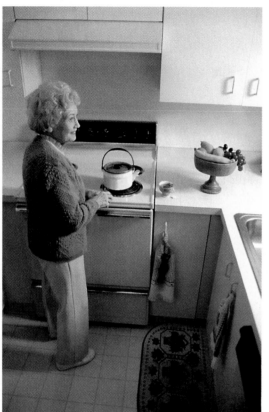

Fig. 3-1. Understand that many residents had to leave familiar places.

- loss of ability to attend services and meetings at their faith communities
- loss of ability to care for themselves

Independence often means not having to rely on others for money, daily routine care, or participation in social activities. **Activities of Daily Living (ADLs)** are the personal care tasks you do every day to care for yourself. People take these activities for granted until they can no longer do them for themselves. ADLs include bathing or showering, dressing, caring for teeth and hair, toileting, eating and drinking, and moving from place to place.

A loss of independence can cause:

- a negative self-image
- anger toward caregivers, others, and self
- feelings of helplessness, sadness, and hopelessness

- feelings of being useless
- increased dependence
- depression

To prevent these feelings, encourage residents to do as much as possible for themselves. Even if it seems easier for you to do things for your residents, allow them to accomplish a task independently. Encourage self-care, regardless of how long it takes or how poorly they are able to do it. Be patient while they do these tasks (Fig. 3-2).

When you assist residents with their ADLs, it is important to provide respect, dignity, and privacy. This includes the following:

- Do not interrupt them while they are in the bathroom.
- Leave the room when they receive or make personal phone calls.
- Respect their private time and personal property.
- Do not interrupt them if they are dressing themselves.
- Encourage them to do things for themselves. Be patient while they do so.
- Be patient while residents choose their clothing. Keep their bodies covered whenever possible when you assist with dressing.

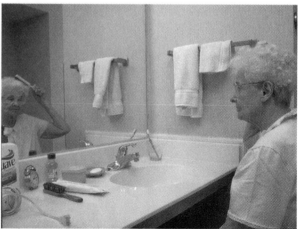

Fig. 3-2. Even if tasks take a long time, encourage residents to do what they can for themselves.

RA Never treat residents as children. They are adults. Encourage them to do self-care without rushing them. Remember that they have the right to refuse care and make their own choices. Maintaining your residents' dignity and independence is not only their legal right, but it is also the proper and ethical way for you to work.

Unit 2: **Identify basic human needs**

People have different genes, physical appearances, cultural backgrounds, ages, and social or financial positions. But all human beings have the same basic physical needs:

- food and water
- protection and shelter
- activity
- sleep and rest
- safety
- comfort, especially freedom from pain

We also have **psychosocial needs**, which involve social interaction, emotions, intellect, and spirituality. Psychosocial needs are not as easy to define as physical needs. However, all human beings have the following psychosocial needs:

- love and affection
- acceptance by others
- security
- self-reliance and independence in daily living
- interaction with other people (Fig. 3-3)
- accomplishments and self-esteem

Our health and well-being are affected by how well our psychosocial needs are met. Frustration and stress occur when our basic needs are not met. This can lead to fear, anxiety, anger, aggression, withdrawal, indifference, and depression.

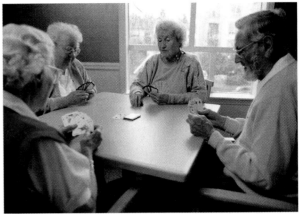

Fig. 3-3. Social interaction is an important psychosocial need.

Abraham Maslow, a researcher of human behavior, wrote about human physical, psychological, and social needs. He arranged these needs into an order of importance. He thought that our physical needs must be met before we can work on meeting our psychological or social needs. His theory is called "Maslow's Hierarchy of Needs" (Fig 3-4).

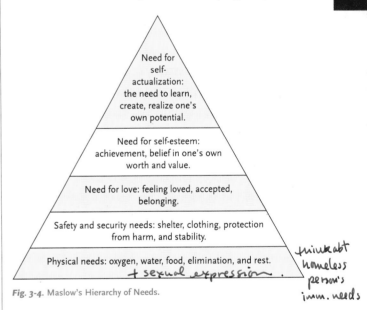

Need for self-actualization: the need to learn, create, realize one's own potential.

Need for self-esteem: achievement, belief in one's own worth and value.

Need for love: feeling loved, accepted, belonging.

Safety and security needs: shelter, clothing, protection from harm, and stability.

Physical needs: oxygen, water, food, elimination, and rest. *+ sexual expression.*

think abt homeless person's imm. needs

Fig. 3-4. Maslow's Hierarchy of Needs.

People continue to have sexual needs throughout their lives (Fig. 3-5). The ability to engage in sexual activity, such as intercourse and masturbation, continues unless a disease or injury occurs. Always knock or announce yourself before entering a resident's room. Listen for a response. If you encounter a sexual situation, your role is to provide privacy.

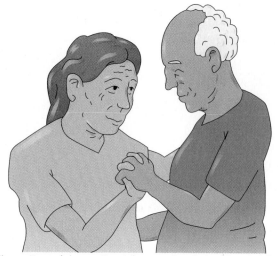

Fig. 3-5. Human beings continue to have sexual needs throughout their lives.

Residents have the right to choose how they express their sexuality. In all age groups, there is a variety of sexual behavior. This is true of your residents also. Do not judge any sexual behavior you see. An attitude that any expression of sexuality by the elderly is disgusting or cute deprives your residents of their right to dignity and respect.

Residents have spiritual needs. You can assist with these needs, too. Ways you can help residents with their spiritual needs include

- If they are religious, encourage participation in religious services.

- Report to the nurse (or social worker) if your resident expresses the desire to see clergy.

- Listen carefully to what your resident says.

- Respect all religious items.

- Respect your resident's decision to participate in, or refrain from, food-related rituals.

- Allow privacy for clergy and visitors.

- If they ask you to do so, read inspirational or sacred materials aloud.

You should never

- try to change someone's religion

- tell a resident his/her belief or religion is wrong

- express judgments about a religious group

- insist a resident join religious activities

- interfere with religious practices

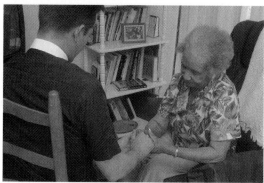

Fig. 3-6. Do not try to change a resident's spiritual beliefs. Be welcoming when they receive a visit from a spiritual leader.

There are many community resources available to help your residents meet their different needs. Some of these resources are:

- Area Agency on Aging

- Ombudsman program

- Alzheimer's Association

- local Hospice organization

- social workers

- resident advocacy organizations

📋 *Surveyors will expect the facility to provide residents with information about community resources—especially those organizations that protect the rights of residents.*

Unit 3: **Identify ways to accommodate cultural differences**

Imagine if there were only one restaurant, one place to worship, or one style of clothing or house. It would be very boring. Luckily, in most developed countries, people have many different cultural backgrounds and religious traditions. You will take care of residents of different backgrounds and traditions other than your own. It is important to respect and value each person as an individual.

Sometimes it is easier to accept different practices or beliefs if you understand a little about them.

There are so many different cultures that they cannot all be listed here. A **culture** is a system of behaviors people learn from the people they grow up and live with. One might talk about American culture being different from Japanese culture. But within American culture there are thousands of different groups with their own cultures: Japanese-Americans, African-Americans, and Native Americans, just to name a few. Even people from a particular region, state, or city can be said to have a different culture (Fig. 3-7). The culture of the south is not the same as the culture of New York City.

Cultural background affects how friendly people are to strangers. It can affect how close they want you to stand to them when talking. Be sensitive to the backgrounds of your residents. You cannot expect to be treated the same way by all your residents. You may have to adjust your behavior around each of your residents. Regardless of their background, you must treat all residents with respect and professionalism.

A resident's primary language may be different from yours. If he or she speaks a different language, an interpreter may be necessary. Take time to learn a few common phrases in a resident's native language. Picture cards and flash cards can assist with communication.

Religious differences also influence the way people behave. Religion can be very important in people's lives, particularly when they are ill or dying. You must respect the religious beliefs and practices of your residents. Do this especially if they are different from your own. Never question your residents' be-

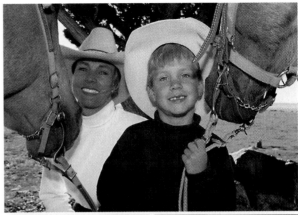
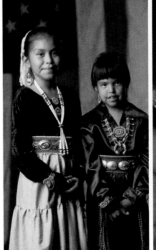
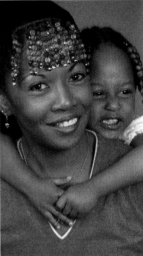

Fig. 3-7. There are many different cultures in the United States.

liefs. Do not discuss your own beliefs with them.

Be aware of practices that affect your work with residents. Many religious beliefs include food restrictions, or rules about what and when followers can eat and drink. For example, Jewish people may not eat any pork. Be aware of any dietary restrictions and honor them. (Food differences will be discussed more in chapter 7.)

Some people's backgrounds may make them less comfortable being touched by others. Be sensitive to your residents' feelings. You must touch residents in order to do your job. However, recognize that some residents feel more comfortable when there is little physical contact. Learn about your residents. Adjust your care to their needs.

Understanding Your Residents

Unit 4: Discuss family roles and their significance in health care

Families are the most important unit within our social system. Families play a huge role in most people's lives (Fig. 3-8). Some examples of family types are listed below.

- Single-parent families include one parent with a child or children.

- Nuclear families include two parents with a child or children.

- Blended families include widowed or divorced parents who have remarried, with children from previous marriages as well as from this marriage.

- Multigenerational families include parents, children, and grandparents.

- Extended families may include aunts, uncles, cousins, or even friends.

- Families may also be made up of unmarried couples of the same sex or opposite sexes, with or without children.

In long-term care, family members help in many ways:

- helping residents make care decisions

- communicating with the care team

- giving support and encouragement

- connecting the resident to the outside world

- offering assurance to dying residents that family memories and traditions will be valued and carried on

Be respectful and nice to friends and family members. Allow privacy for visits. After any visitor leaves, observe the effect the visit had on the resident. Report any noticeable effects to the nurse. Some residents have good relationships with their families, while others do not. If you notice any abusive behavior from a visitor towards a resident, report it immediately to the nurse.

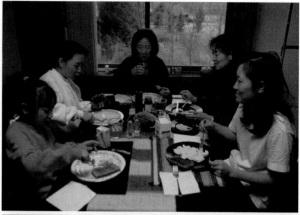

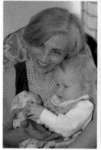 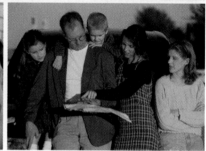

Fig. 3-8. Families come in all shapes and sizes.

RA *The facility has a contract with the resident to provide care 24 hours a day. Families have every right to expect quality care to continue when they cannot be with their loved one. Your obligation includes the family's concerns.*

Families are great sources of information for the resident's personal preferences, history, diet, rituals, and routines. Take time to ask them questions. Families often seek out nursing assistants because they are closest to the residents. This is an important responsibility. Show families that you have time for them too. Communicate with them, but do not discuss a resident's care with friends or family members. Listen if they want to talk. Refer questions regarding care to your supervisor.

Unit 5: Describe the stages of human development

Everyone will go through the same stages of development during his or her life. However, no two people will follow the exact same pattern or rate of development. Each resident must be treated as an individual and a whole person who is growing and developing. They should not be treated as someone who is merely ill or disabled.

Infancy, Birth to Twelve Months

Infants grow and develop very quickly. In one year a baby moves from total dependence to the relative independence of moving around, communicating basic needs, and feeding himself.

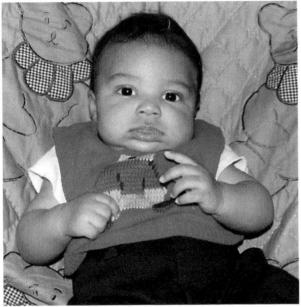

Fig. 3-9. An infant's physical development moves from the head down.

Physical development in infancy moves from the head down. For example, infants gain control over the muscles of the neck before they are able to control the muscles in their shoulders. Control over muscles in the trunk area, such as the shoulder, develops before control of arms and legs (Fig. 3-9).

Childhood

The Toddler Period, Ages One to Three

During the toddler years, children gain independence. One part of this independence is new control over their bodies. Toddlers learn to speak, gain coordination of their limbs, and learn to control their bladders and bowels (Fig. 3-10).

Toddlers assert their new independence by exploring further and further from the caregiver. Poisons and other hazards, such as sharp objects, must be locked away.

Psychologically, toddlers learn that they are individuals, separate from their parents. Children of this age may try to control their parents. They may try to get what they want by throwing tantrums, whining, or refusing to cooperate. This is a key time for parents to establish rules and standards.

The Preschool Years, Ages Three to Six

Children in their preschool years develop skills that will help them become more independent and have social relationships (Fig. 3-11). They develop vocabulary and language skills. They learn to play cooperatively in groups. They become more physically coordinated, and learn to care for themselves. Preschoolers also develop ways of relating to family members, and they begin to learn right from wrong.

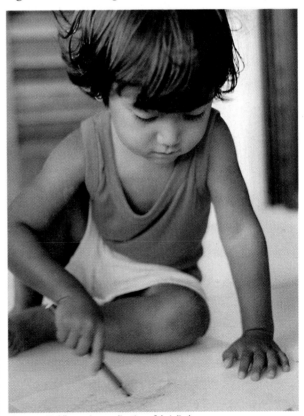

Fig. 3-10. Toddlers gain coordination of their limbs.

Understanding Your Residents

School-Age Children, Ages Six to Twelve

From ages six to about twelve years, children's development is centered on **cognitive** (developing thinking and learning skills) and social development. As children enter school, they also explore the environment around them and relate to other children through games, peer groups, and classroom activities. In these years, children learn to get along with each other. They also begin to behave in a way that is common among their sex, and they develop a conscience, morals, and self-esteem.

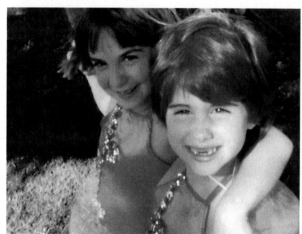

Fig. 3-11. Children in preschool years develop social relationships.

Adolescence

Puberty

During puberty secondary sex characteristics, such as body hair appear. Also, reproductive organs begin to function due to the secretion of the reproductive hormones. The onset of puberty occurs between the ages of ten and sixteen for girls and twelve and fourteen for boys.

Adolescence, Ages Twelve to Eighteen

Many teenagers have a difficult time adapting to the changes that occur in their bodies after puberty. Peer acceptance is important to them. Because they see images of perfection in the media, adolescents may be afraid that they are unattractive or even abnormal (Fig. 3-12).

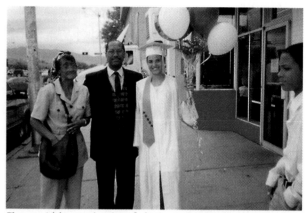

Fig. 3-12. Adolescence is a time of adapting to change.

This concern for body image and acceptance, combined with changing hormones that influence moods, can cause adolescents to swing rapidly from one mood to another. They remain dependent on their parents and yet need to express themselves socially and sexually. This causes conflict and stress. Social interaction between members of the opposite sex becomes very important.

Adulthood

Young Adulthood, Ages Eighteen to Forty

By the age of eighteen, most young adults have stopped growing. Adopting a healthy lifestyle in these years can make life better now and prevent health problems in later adulthood. Psychological and social development continues, however. The developmental tasks of these years include

- selecting an appropriate education and an occupation or career

- selecting a mate (Fig. 3-13)

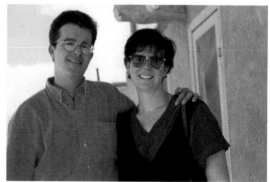

Fig. 3-13. Young adulthood often involves finding long-term mates.

- learning to live with a mate or others

- raising children

- developing a satisfying sex life

Middle Adulthood: Forty to Sixty-five Years

In general, people in middle adulthood are more comfortable and stable than they were in previous stages. Many of their major life decisions have already been made. In the early years of middle adulthood people sometimes experience a "mid-life crisis." This is a period of unrest centered on an unconscious desire for change and fulfillment of unmet goals.

Late Adulthood: Sixty-five Years and Older

Persons in late adulthood must adjust to the effects of aging. These effects or changes can include the loss of physical strength and health, the death of loved ones, retirement, and preparation for their own death. Although the developmental tasks of this age appear to deal entirely with loss, the solutions to these problems often involve new relationships, friendships, and interests.

Because later adulthood covers an age range of as many as 25 to 35 years, people in this age category can have very different capabilities, depending on their health. Some 70-year-old people still enjoy active sports, while others are not active (Fig. 3-14). Many 85-year-old people can still live alone, though others may live with family members or in nursing homes. Generalizations about older people are often false. They create prejudices against the elderly that are as unfair as prejudices against racial, ethnic, or religious groups.

On television or in the movies older people are often shown as helpless, lonely, disabled, slow, forgetful, dependent, or inactive. However, research shows that most older people are active and engaged in work, volunteer activities, and learning and exercise

programs. Aging is a normal process, not a disease. Most older people live independent lives and do not need assistance (Fig. 3-15).

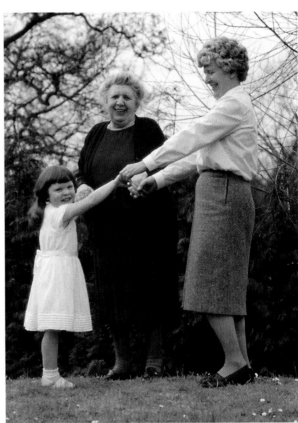

Fig. 3-14. Older adults often remain active and engaged.

As a nursing assistant you will spend much of your time working with elderly residents. You must know what is true about aging and what is not true. While aging causes many physical, psychological, and social changes, *normal changes of aging do not mean an older person must become dependent, ill, or inactive.* Knowing normal changes of aging from signs of illness or disability will allow you to better help your elderly residents.

Normal changes of aging include the following:

- skin is thinner, drier and more fragile

- muscles are not as strong

- senses of vision, hearing, taste and smell change

- heart is less efficient

- appetite changes
- more frequent elimination
- production of hormones changes
- weakened immunity
- mild forgetfulness
- lifestyle changes

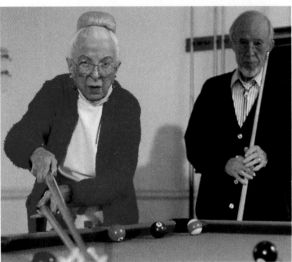

Fig. 3-15. Most older people lead active lives.

There are also changes that are NOT considered normal changes of aging and should be reported to the nurse. These include

- signs of depression
- loss of ability to think logically
- poor nutritional status
- shortness of breath
- incontinence

Keep in mind that this is not a complete list. *Your job includes reporting any change, normal or not.*

Unit 6: **Discuss the needs of people with developmental disabilities**

A small number of people you will care for are developmentally disabled. A developmental disability is a chronic condition that restricts physical or mental ability. Their care will depend on the type and the extent of the disability. A person may not be able to perform certain activities, including activities of daily living (ADLs). A person's ability to communicate may be affected. His or her ability to learn may be limited as well. Many persons with developmental disabilities require special care, treatment or other services for long periods of time or throughout their lives.

Mental retardation is the most common developmental disorder. Approximately 1% of the general population has mental retardation. It is neither a disease nor a psychiatric illness. People with mental retardation develop at a below-average rate. They have below-average mental functioning. They experience difficulty in learning and may have problems adjusting socially.

People who are developmentally disabled require the same respect, preservation of dignity, and quality care as your other residents.

GUIDELINES
Developmentally Disabled Residents

- Treat them as adults, regardless of the behavior they exhibit.
- Praise and encourage often.
- Repeat words you use to make sure they understand.
- Be patient.

Unit 7: **Explain how to care for dying residents**

Death can occur suddenly and without warning, or it can be expected. Older people, or people with terminal illnesses, may have time to prepare for death. A **terminal illness** is a disease or condition that will eventually cause death. Preparing for death is a process that involves the dying person's emotions and behavior.

Dr. Elisabeth Kubler-Ross researched and wrote about the process of dying. Her book, *On Death and Dying*, describes five stages that dying people and their families or friends may experience before death. These five stages are described below.

Denial. People in the denial stage may refuse to believe they are dying. They often believe a mistake has been made.

Anger. Once they start to face the possibility of their death, people become angry that they are the ones who are dying.

Bargaining. Once people have begun to believe that they are dying, they may make promises to God or somehow try to bargain for their recovery.

Depression. As dying people become physically weaker and symptoms of their illness get worse, they may become deeply sad or depressed.

Acceptance. Some people who are dying are eventually able to accept death and prepare for it. They may make plans for their last days or for the ceremonies that may follow.

Some residents will have advance directives, or they may create them before they die. **Advance directives** are documents that allow people to choose what kind of medical care they wish to have if they are unable to make those decisions themselves. Be familiar with advance directives. One example is a "Do Not Resuscitate" (DNR) order. This is a healthcare order that tells medical professionals not to perform CPR. An advance directive can also name someone else to make medical decisions for a person if that person becomes disabled. A Living Will is one example of this.

As with dying, grieving is an individual process. No two people will grieve in exactly the same way. Clergy, counselors, or social workers can provide help for people who are grieving (Fig. 3-16). Family members or friends may have any of the following reactions to the death of a loved one.

- shock
- denial
- anger
- guilt
- regret
- sadness
- loneliness

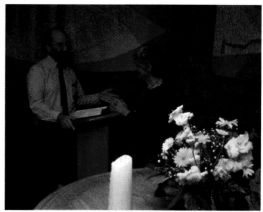

Fig. 3-16. Some people will speak with clergy to help them deal with their grief.

Death is a very sensitive topic. Many people find it hard to discuss death. Feelings and attitudes about death can be influenced by many factors, such as

- previous experiences with death
- personality type
- religious beliefs
- cultural background

RA *When a resident is dying, be considerate and respectful. Do not avoid a dying resident. Listening may be one of the most important things you can do for a resident who is dying. Provide privacy for visits from family and friends.*

Common signs of approaching death include the following:

- blurred and failing vision

- unfocused eyes

- impaired speech

- diminished sense of touch

- loss of movement, muscle tone, and feeling

- a rising or below-normal body temperature

- decreasing blood pressure

- weak pulse that is abnormally slow or rapid

- slow, irregular respirations or rapid, shallow respirations

- a "rattling" or "gurgling" sound as the person breathes

- cold, pale skin

- mottling, spotting, or blotching of skin caused by poor circulation

- perspiration

- incontinence

- disorientation or confusion

GUIDELINES
Caring for the Dying Resident

- **Diminished senses**. Keep room softly lighted without glare. Hearing is usually the last sense to leave the body, so speak in a normal tone. Observe body language to anticipate a resident's needs (Fig. 3-17).

- **Care of the mouth**. Give mouth care frequently. If the resident is unconscious, give mouth care every two hours. Apply lubricant, such as lip balm, to lips.

- **Skin care**. Give bed baths and incontinent care as needed. Bathe perspiring residents often. Sheets and clothes should be changed for comfort. Keep sheets wrinkle-free. Skin care to prevent pressure sores is important. (More on pressure sores is in chapter 5.)

- **Comfort**. Observe for signs of pain. Frequent changes of position, back massage, skin care, mouth care and proper body alignment may help. Report any signs of pain.

- **Environment**. Display favorite objects and photographs for resident. Make sure room is appropriately lighted and well ventilated.

- **Emotional and spiritual support**. Listen to resident if he or she wishes to talk. Touch is important. Some residents may seek spiritual comfort from clergy.

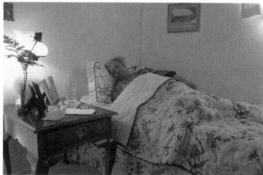

Fig. 3-17. Keep a dying resident's room softly lighted without glare.

♥ *After death, the eyelids may be partially open with the eyes in a fixed stare. The mouth may fall open as the jaw muscles relax. Sometimes the person may be incontinent as the muscles relax. Even though these things are a normal part of death, they can be frightening. Inform the nurse immediately to help confirm the death.*

GUIDELINES
Postmortem Care

Your facility's guidelines should be followed. They may include the following:

- Bathe the body. Be gentle to avoid bruising. Place drainage pads where needed.

- Do not remove any tubes or other equipment.

- Put dentures back in the mouth and close the mouth. If not possible, place dentures in denture cup near head.

- Close the eyes carefully.

- Position the body on the back with legs straight, arms folded across the abdomen. Put a small pillow under the head.

- Follow facility policy on personal items. Check to see if you should remove jewelry. Always have a witness if personal items are removed or given to a family member. Document what was given to whom.

- Document according to your facility's policy.

- Remember to respect the wishes of family and friends. Be sensitive to their needs after death occurs. Only perform assigned tasks.

Unit 8: Define the goals of a hospice program

Hospice care is the term used for the special care that a dying person needs. Hospice care may be provided in a hospital, a special care facility, or in the home. A hospice can be any location where a person who is dying is treated with dignity by caregivers who are specially trained to provide for their physical, emotional, social, and spiritual needs.

Hospice often includes treatment for pain. Residents who are dying also need to feel some independence for as long as possible. Caregivers should allow residents to retain as much control over their lives as possible. Eventually, caregivers may have to meet all of the resident's basic needs.

Other attitudes and skills useful when providing hospice care include the following:

- Develop and explore your own personal feelings and strengths about death and dying.

- Ask family members or friends how you can be of help.

- Be a good listener, and do not feel obligated to respond.

- Recognize that some persons wish to be alone with their dying loved ones.

- Respect privacy and independence.

I have the right to:

be treated as a living human being until I die.

maintain a sense of hopefulness, however changing its focus may be.

be cared for by those who can maintain a sense of hopefulness, however changing this might be.

express my feelings and emotions about my approaching death in my own way.

participate in decisions concerning my care.

expect continuing medical and nursing attentions even though "cure" goals must be changed to "comfort" goals.

to die alone.

be free from pain.

have my questions answered honestly.

not be deceived.

have help from and for my family in accepting my death.

die in peace and dignity.

retain my individuality and not be judged for my decisions which may be contrary to beliefs of others.

discuss and enlarge my religious and/or spiritual experiences, whatever these may mean to others.

expect that the sanctity of the human body will be respected after death.

be cared for by caring, sensitive, knowledgeable people who will attempt to understand my needs and will be able to gain some satisfaction in helping me face my death.

Fig. 3-18. The Dying Person's Bill of Rights.

In long-term care, goals include a focus on residents getting healthier, or helping the resident to care for him or herself as much as possible. In hospice care, however, the goals of care are the comfort and dignity of the resident (Fig. 3-18). This is an important difference. You will need to adjust your mindset when caring for hospice residents. Focus on relieving their pain and making them comfortable, rather than on teaching them to care for themselves.

Understanding Your Residents

FOUR

Body Systems

Our bodies are organized into body systems. Each system has conditions under which it works best. **Homeostasis** is the name for the condition in which all of the body's systems are working their best. To be in homeostasis, our body's **metabolism**, or physical and chemical processes, must be operating at a steady level. When disease or injury occur, the body's metabolism is disturbed. Homeostasis is lost.

Each system in the body has its own unique structure and function, or job. There are also normal, age-related changes for each body system. You need to understand what a normal change of aging is for a particular body system. This will help you better recognize any abnormal changes in your residents. We have also included tips on how you can assist your residents with their normal changes of aging.

Body systems can be broken down in different ways. In this book we divide the human body into ten body systems.

1. Integumentary, or skin
2. Musculoskeletal
3. Nervous
4. Circulatory or cardiovascular
5. Respiratory
6. Urinary
7. Gastrointestinal or digestive
8. Endocrine
9. Reproductive
10. Immune and Lymphatic

Body systems are made up of organs. Organs are made up of tissues. Tissues are made up of groups of cells that perform a similar task. For example, in the circulatory system, the heart is one of the organs. It is made up of tissues and cells. Cells are the building blocks of our bodies. Living cells divide, develop, and die, renewing the tissues and organs of our body.

Unit 1: **Describe the integumentary system**

The largest organ and system in the body is the skin, a natural protective covering or integument. Skin prevents injury to internal organs. It also protects the body against entry of bacteria or germs. Skin also prevents the loss of too much water, which is essential to life. Skin is made up of tissues and **glands**, which are structures that secrete fluids (Fig. 4-1).

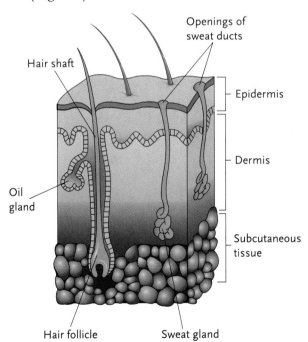

Openings of sweat ducts
Hair shaft
Epidermis
Oil gland
Dermis
Subcutaneous tissue
Hair follicle
Sweat gland

Fig. 4-1. Cross-section showing details of the integumentary system.

The skin is also a *sense* organ that feels heat, cold, pain, touch, and pressure. Body temperature is regulated in the skin, which has blood vessels that **dilate**, or widen, when the outside temperature is too high. This brings more blood to the body surface to cool it off. The same blood vessels **constrict**, or close, when the outside temperature is too cold. By restricting the amount of blood reaching the skin, the blood vessels help the body retain heat.

Normal changes of aging include

- skin gets thinner and more fragile, so it is more easily damaged
- skin dries and is less elastic
- hair thins and turns gray
- wrinkles and brown spots, or liver spots, appear
- protective fatty tissue gets thinner, so person feels colder
- fingernails and toenails thicken and become tougher

How You Can Help: Nursing Assistant's Role

Keep the resident's skin clean and dry. Use lotions as ordered for moisture. Layer clothing and bed covers for additional warmth. Keep sheets wrinkle-free. Provide careful nail care. If you are allowed to clip fingernails, do so with extreme caution. Encourage fluids.

INTEGUMENTARY SYSTEM:
Observing and Reporting

Observe and report the following signs and symptoms:

- rashes or scales
- bruising
- cuts, boils, sores, wounds, abrasions
- changes in color or moistness/dryness
- swelling
- scalp or hair changes
- skin that appears different from normal or that has changed

COMMON DISORDERS
Integumentary System

- Pressure sores, or decubitus ulcers (See chapter 5.)

Unit 2: Describe the musculoskeletal system

Muscles, bones, ligaments, tendons, and cartilage give the body shape and structure. They work together to allow the body to move (Fig. 4-2). Exercise is important for improving and maintaining physical and mental health. For residents who are ill or elderly and are unable to exercise much, range of motion (ROM) exercises can help. ROM exercises can prevent problems related to immobility. These include a loss of self-esteem, depression, pneumonia, urinary tract infection, constipation, blood clots, dulling of the senses, and muscle atrophy or contractures. **Contractures** are the painful stiffening of a joint and muscle. (See chapter 9 for more information on ROM exercises.)

Normal changes of aging include

- muscles weaken and lose tone
- body movement slows
- joints become less flexible
- bones lose density and become more brittle, making them easy to break
- gradual loss of height

OBSERVING AND REPORTING
Musculoskeletal System

Observe and report the following signs and symptoms:

- changes in ability to perform routine movements and activities
- any changes in residents' ability to perform ROM exercises
- pain during movement
- any new or increased swelling of joints
- white, shiny, red, or warm areas over a joint
- bruising
- aches and pains residents report to you

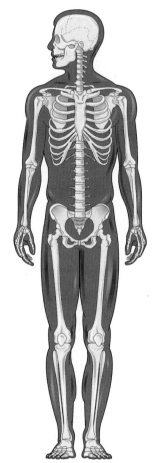

Fig. 4-2. The skeleton is composed of 206 bones that help movement and protect organs.

How You Can Help: Nursing Assistant's Role

Falls can cause life-threatening complications, including fractures. Prevent falls by keeping items out of the resident's path. Keep furniture in the same place. Keep walker or cane where resident can easily get to it. Encourage regular movement and self-care. Assist with range of motion (ROM) exercises as needed. Encourage the person to perform as many ADLs as possible.

COMMON DISORDERS
Musculoskeletal System

- Fractures
- Osteoporosis

cd Arthritis

cd Contractures

For more information on these disorders, see chapter 8.

Unit 3: **Describe the nervous system**

The nervous system is the control center and message center of the body. It controls and coordinates all body functions. The nervous system also senses and interprets information from the environment outside the human body (Fig. 4-3).

Normal changes of aging include:

- slower responses and reflexes

- decrease in sensitivity of nerve endings in skin

- some memory loss, more often with short-term memory

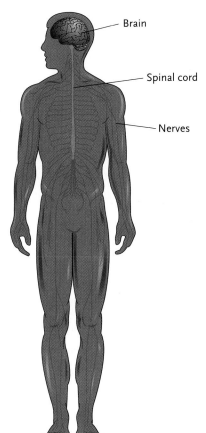

Fig. 4-3. The nervous system includes the brain, spinal cord, and nerves throughout the body.

OBSERVING AND REPORTING
Central Nervous System

Observe and report the following signs and symptoms:

O&R fatigue or any pain with movement or exercise

O&R shaking or trembling

O&R inability to speak clearly

O&R inability to move one side of body

O&R disturbance or changes in vision or hearing

O&R changes in eating patterns and/or fluid intake

O&R difficulty swallowing

O&R bowel and bladder changes

O&R depression or mood changes

O&R memory loss or confusion

O&R violent behavior

O&R any unusual or unexplained change in behavior

O&R decreased ability to perform ADLs

COMMON DISORDERS
Central Nervous System

cd Dementias, including Alzheimer's disease and Parkinson's disease*

cd Cerebrovascular accident (CVA), or stroke*

cd Multiple Sclerosis*

cd Epilepsy

cd Cerebral Palsy

cd Head and spinal cord injuries*

Body Systems

* For more information on these disorders, see chapter 8.

The Nervous System: Sense Organs

The eyes, ears, nose, tongue, and skin are the body's major sense organs. They are considered part of the central nervous system because they receive impulses from the environment. They relay these impulses to nerves (Fig. 4-4 and Fig. 4-5).

Normal changes of aging include

- reduced vision and hearing (sense of balance may be affected)

- decreased sense of taste and ability to smell

- decreased sensitivity to heat and cold

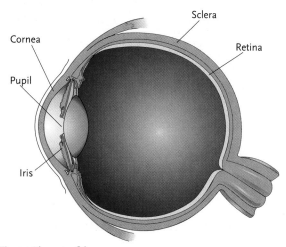

Fig. 4-4. The parts of the eye.

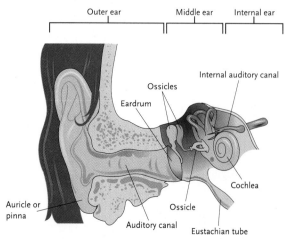

Fig. 4-5. The outer ear, middle ear, and inner ear are the three main divisions of the ear.

How You Can Help: Nursing Assistant's Role

Encourage the use of eyeglasses and hearing aides and keep them clean. Speak slowly and clearly; do not shout.

OBSERVING AND REPORTING
Eyes and Ears

Observe and report the following signs and symptoms:

- changes in vision or hearing

- signs of infection

- dizziness

- resident complaints of pain in eyes or ears

COMMON DISORDERS
Eyes and Ears

- Cataracts

- Glaucoma

- Deafness

Unit 4: Describe the circulatory or cardiovascular system

The circulatory system is made up of the heart, blood vessels, and blood. The heart pumps blood through the blood vessels to the cells. The blood carries food, oxygen, and other substances cells need to function properly (Fig. 4-6).

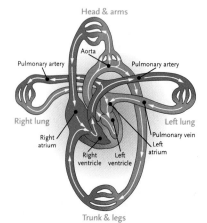

Fig. 4-6. The flow of blood through the heart.

The circulatory system performs the following major functions:

- supplying food, oxygen, and hormones to cells

- producing and supplying infection-fighting blood cells

- removing waste products from cells

- controlling body temperature

Normal changes of aging include

- loss of heart muscle strength

- narrowed blood vessels

- decreased blood flow

How You Can Help: Nursing Assistant's Role

Encourage movement and exercise. Allow enough time to complete these activities. Prevent person from becoming too tired. Keep legs and feet warm.

Observe and report the following signs and symptoms:

- changes in pulse rate

- weakness, fatigue

- loss of ability to perform activities of daily living (ADLs)

- swelling of hands and feet

- pale or blue appearance of hands, feet, or lips

- chest pain

- weight gain

- shortness of breath, changes in breathing patterns, inability to catch their breath

- severe headache

- inactivity (which can lead to circulatory problems)

- Hardening and narrowing of the blood vessels

- Myocardial infarction (MI), or heart attack*

- Angina pectoris*

- Hypertension, or high blood pressure*

- Congestive heart failure*

- Peripheral vascular disease*

* For more information on these disorders, see chapter 8.

Unit 5: **Describe the respiratory system**

Respiration, the body taking in oxygen and removing carbon dioxide, involves breathing in (**inspiration**), and breathing out (**expiration**). The lungs accomplish this process (Fig. 4-7).

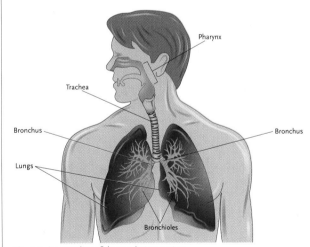

Fig. 4-7. An overview of the respiratory system.

The respiratory system of the body has two functions:

1. It brings oxygen into the body.

2. It eliminates carbon dioxide produced as the body uses oxygen.

Normal changes of aging include

- loss of lung strength

- decreased lung capacity
- decreased oxygen in the blood
- weakened voice

How You Can Help: Nursing Assistant's Role

Encourage the person to get out of bed as often as possible. Encourage exercise and regular movement. Encourage and assist with deep breathing exercises.

OBSERVING AND REPORTING
Respiratory System

Observe and report the following signs and symptoms:

- change in respiratory rate
- shallow breathing or breathing through pursed lips
- coughing or wheezing
- nasal congestion or discharge
- sore throat, difficulty swallowing, or swollen tonsils
- the need to sit after mild exertion
- the need to rest on two pillows
- pale or bluish color of the lips and arms and legs
- pain in the chest area
- discolored **sputum**, or the fluid a person coughs up (green, yellow, blood-tinged, or gray)

COMMON DISORDERS
Respiratory System

- Asthma*
- Upper respiratory infection (URI), or a cold
- Bronchitis*
- Pneumonia*
- Emphysema*
- Lung cancer
- Tuberculosis
- Chronic Obstructive Pulmonary Disease*

* For more information on these disorders, see chapter 8.

Unit 6: **Describe the urinary system**

The urinary system has two vital functions:

1. Through urine, it eliminates waste products created by the cells.
2. It maintains water balance in the body.

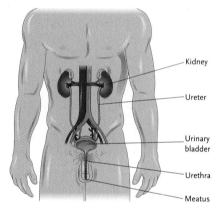

Fig. 4-8. The male urinary system.

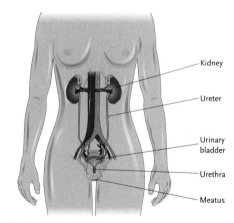

Fig. 4-9. The female urinary system.

Normal changes of aging include

- reduced ability of kidneys to filter blood
- weakened bladder muscle tone
- bladder holds less urine, causing more frequent urination
- bladder may not empty completely, causing more susceptibility to infection

How You Can Help:
Nursing Assistant's Role

Encourage residents to drink fluids. Offer frequent trips to the bathroom. If person is incontinent, do not show frustration or anger. Keep person clean and dry.

OBSERVING AND REPORTING
Urinary System

Observe and report the following signs and symptoms:

- weight loss or gain

- swelling in the upper or the lower extremities

- painful urination or burning during urination

- changes in the characteristics of urine, such as cloudiness, odor, or color

- changes in frequency and amount of urination

- swelling in the abdominal/bladder area

- resident complaining that bladder feels full or painful

- incontinence/dribbling

- pain in the kidney or back/flank region

- inadequate fluid intake

COMMON DISORDERS
Urinary System

- Urinary tract infection (UTI), or cystitis

- Calculi (kidney stones)

- Nephritis

- Renovascular hypertension

- Chronic kidney failure

Unit 7: **Describe the gastrointestinal or digestive system**

The gastrointestinal system, also called the digestive system, has two functions:

1. Digestion. The process of changing food so that it can be absorbed into the cells.

2. Elimination. The process of expelling solid wastes that are not absorbed into the cells.

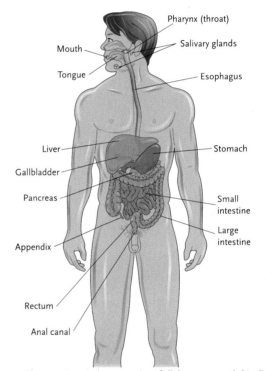

Fig. 4-10. The gastrointestinal tract consists of all the organs needed to digest food and process waste.

Normal changes of aging include

- decrease of saliva and digestive fluids

- difficulty chewing and swallowing

- decrease in absorption of vitamins and minerals

- less efficient process of digestion; more frequent constipation

How You Can Help:
Nursing Assistant's Role

Encourage fluids and nutritious, appealing meals. Allow time to eat. Make mealtime enjoyable. Provide good oral care. Make sure dentures fit properly and are cleaned regularly. Encourage daily bowel movements. Give person opportunity to have a bowel movement around the same time each day.

Body Systems

Gastrointestinal System

Observe and report the following signs and symptoms:

- difficulty swallowing or chewing (including denture problems, tooth pain, or mouth sores)

- fecal incontinence (losing control of bowels)

- weight gain/weight loss

- anorexia (loss of appetite)

- abdominal pain and cramping

- diarrhea

- nausea and vomiting (especially vomitus that looks like coffee grounds)

- constipation

- gas

- hiccoughs, belching

- abnormally-colored stool (bloody, black, or hard)

- heartburn

- poor nutritional intake

Gastrointestinal System

- Peptic ulcers

- Hepatitis

- Ulcerative colitis

- Colorectal cancer

- Hemorrhoids

Unit 8: Describe the endocrine system

The endocrine system is made up of glands that secrete hormones. **Hormones** are chemicals that control many of the organs and body systems (Fig. 4-11). They are carried in blood to the organs, where they do the following:

- maintain homeostasis

- influence growth and development

- regulate levels of sugar in the blood

- regulate levels of calcium in the bones

- determine how fast cells burn food for energy

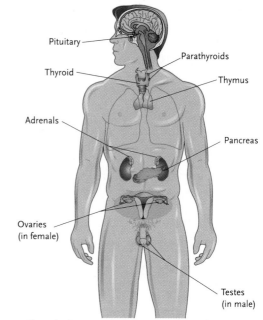

Fig. 4-11. The endocrine system includes organs that produce hormones that regulate body processes.

Normal changes of aging include:

- decrease in levels of hormones, such as estrogen and progesterone

- less production of insulin

- less able to handle stress

How You Can Help:
Nursing Assistant's Role

*Encourage proper nutrition. Remove or reduce stressors. **Stressors** are anything that causes stress. Offer encouragement and listen to the person.*

Endocrine System

Many endocrine illnesses can be treated with hormone supplements. These supplements must be given very precisely. For example, too much insulin administered to a diabetic can cause the sudden start of insulin shock.

Observe and report the following symptoms:

- headache*
- weakness*
- blurred vision*
- dizziness*
- hunger*
- irritability*
- sweating/excessive perspiration*
- change in "normal" behavior*
- weight gain/weight loss
- loss of appetite/increased appetite
- increased thirst
- frequent urination
- dry skin
- sluggishness or fatigue
- increased confusion
- hyperactivity

* indicates signs and symptoms that should be reported immediately

COMMON DISORDERS
Endocrine System

- Hyperthyroidism
- Hypothyroidism
- Diabetes Mellitus*

* For more information, see chapter 8.

Unit 9: **Describe the reproductive system**

The reproductive system is made up of the reproductive organs, which are different in men and women (Fig. 4-12 and Fig. 4-13). The function of the reproductive system is to allow human beings to **reproduce**, or create new human life. Reproduction begins when a man's and woman's sex cells (sperm and ovum) join. These sex cells are formed in the male and female sex glands. These sex glands are called the gonads.

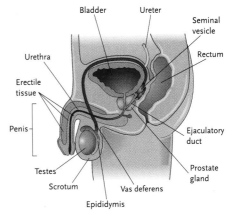

Fig. 4-12. The male reproductive system.

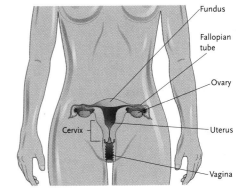

Fig. 4-13. The female reproductive system.

Normal changes of aging include

Female:

- menstruation ends
- decrease in estrogen leads to loss of calcium, causing brittle bones and, potentially, osteoporosis
- drying and thinning of the vaginal walls

Male:

- decrease in sperm production
- enlargement of the prostate gland

How You Can Help:
Nursing Assistant's Role

Sexual needs continue as people age. Provide privacy whenever necessary for sexual activity and respect your residents' sexual needs. Never make fun of or judge any sexual behavior.

RA *Residents have the right to sexual freedom and expression. Residents have the right to privacy and to meet their sexual needs.*

Body Systems

Reproductive System

Observe and report the following signs and symptoms:

- discomfort or difficulty with urination
- discharge from the penis or vagina
- swelling of the genitals
- changes in menstruation
- blood in urine or stool
- breast changes, including size, shape, lumps, or discharge from the nipple
- presence of sores on the genitals
- resident reports of impotence, or inability of male to have sexual intercourse
- resident reports of painful intercourse

Reproductive System

- Breast, prostate, and ovary cancer
- Vaginitis

Unit 10: **Describe the lymphatic and immune systems**

The lymphatic system removes excess fluids and waste products from the body's tissues and helps the immune system fight infection (Fig. 4-14).

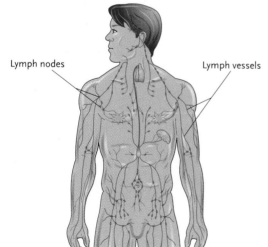

Lymph nodes

Lymph vessels

Fig. 4-14. Lymph nodes work to fight infection and are located throughout the body.

The immune system protects the body from disease-causing bacteria, viruses, and organisms. The immune system protects the body in two ways:

1. Nonspecific immunity protects the body from disease in general.

2. Specific immunity protects against a particular disease that is invading the body at a given time.

Normal changes of aging include

- increased risk of all types of infections
- decreased response to vaccines

How You Can Help:
Nursing Assistant's Role

Follow rules for preventing infection. Wash hands often. Keep the person's environment clean to prevent infection. Encourage and assist with good personal hygiene. Encourage proper nutrition and fluid intake.

Lymphatic System

Observe and report the following symptom:

- swelling of the lymph nodes

Immune System

- Observe and report the following signs and symptoms:
- recurring infections (such as fevers and diarrhea)
- swelling of the lymph nodes
- increased fatigue

Immune System

- HIV/AIDS*
- Lymphoma

* For more information, see chapter 8.

FIVE

Personal Care Skills

Unit 1: Explain personal care of residents

You will assist residents every day with personal care tasks. This includes such activities as bathing, perineal care, mouth care, shampooing and combing hair, nail care, shaving, and dressing. These activities are often referred to as AM care or PM care. This refers to the time of day they are performed.

AM care includes the following:

- offering a bedpan or urinal or assisting the resident to the bathroom
- assisting the resident to wash face and hands
- performing mouth care before or after breakfast depending upon the resident's preference

PM care includes the following:

- offering a bedpan or urinal or assisting the resident to the bathroom
- assisting the resident to wash face and hands
- providing a snack (if allowed)
- performing mouth care
- giving a back rub (if allowed)

How you assist residents with personal care is essential to promoting independence and dignity. Which skills you assist with and how much help you provide will be different for each resident. It depends on a resident's ability to do self-care and/or his or her physical or mental limitations. For example, a resi-

Personal Care Skills

dent who has recently had a stroke will need more assistance with personal care than a resident who has a broken foot that is almost healed.

Personal care is a very private experience. It may be embarrassing for some residents. You must be professional when assisting with these tasks. Before you begin any task, explain to the resident exactly what you will be doing. Ask if he or she would like to use the bathroom or bedpan first. Provide the resident with privacy. Let him or her make as many decisions as possible about when, where, and how a procedure is done (Fig. 5-1). This promotes dignity and independence. Encourage a resident to do as much as he or she is able to do while providing care.

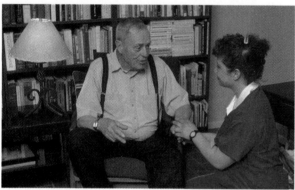

Fig 5-1. Let the resident make as many decisions as possible about the personal care you will perform.

During personal care, observe residents for any problems or changes that have occurred. Personal care offers you an opportunity to talk with residents. Some residents will discuss feelings and concerns with you. You can also observe a resident's environment. Look for physical and mental changes, as well as unsafe or unhealthy surroundings. Report these to the nurse.

If the resident appears tired, stop and take a short rest. Never rush him or her. After care, always ask if the resident would like anything else. Leave the resident's environment clean and tidy. Make sure call light is within reach and bed is left in its lowest position.

OBSERVING AND REPORTING
Personal Care

- skin-color, temperature, reddened areas (more information listed in Unit 7)
- mobility
- flexibility
- comfort level, or any complaints of pain or discomfort
- strength and the ability to perform self-care and ADLs
- mental and emotional state
- resident complaints

Unit 2: **Describe guidelines for assisting with bathing**

Bathing promotes good health and well-being. It removes perspiration, dirt, oil, and dead skin cells that collect on the skin. For bed-bound residents, bed baths will move arms and legs, increasing body movement and circulation. Bathing provides a great opportunity to observe a resident's skin.

GUIDELINES
Bathing

- The face, hands, underarms, and perineum should be washed every day. The **perineum** is the area between the genitals and anus. A complete bath or shower can be taken every other day or even less frequently.

- Older skin produces less perspiration and oil. Elderly people whose skin is dry and fragile should bathe only once or twice a week. This prevents further dryness.

- Use only products approved by the facility or that the resident prefers.

- Before any bathing task, make sure the room is warm enough.

- Before bathing, make sure the water temperature is safe and comfortable.

Ⓖ Gather supplies before giving a bath so a resident is not left alone.

Ⓖ Keep a record of the bathing schedule for each resident. Follow the care plan.

Giving a complete bed bath

Equipment: bath blanket, bath basin, soap, bath thermometer, 2-4 washcloths, 2-4 bath towels, clean gown or clothes, gloves, lotion, deodorant, orange-wood stick or emery board

1. **Wash hands.**
   Provides for infection control.

2. **Identify yourself to resident by name. Address resident by name.**
   Resident has right to know identity of his or her caregiver. Addressing resident by name shows respect and establishes correct identification.

3. **Explain procedure to resident, speaking clearly, slowly, and directly, maintaining face-to-face contact whenever possible.**
   Promotes understanding and independence.

4. **Provide for resident's privacy during procedure with curtain, screen, or door.**
   Maintains resident's right to privacy and dignity.

5. **Adjust bed to a safe working level, usually waist high.**
   Prevents injury to you and to resident.

6. **Adjust position of side rails throughout procedure to ensure resident safety at all times.**

7. **Remove or fold back top bedding, keeping resident covered with bath blanket (or top sheet) (Fig. 5-2).**

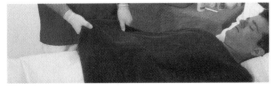

Fig. 5-2.

8. **Test water temperature with thermometer or your wrist and ensure it is safe. Water temperature should be 110° to 115° F because it cools quickly. Have resident check water temperature. Adjust if necessary.**
   Resident's sense of touch may be different than yours; therefore, resident is best able to identify a comfortable water temperature.

9. **If resident has open lesions or wounds, put on gloves.**
   Protects you from coming into contact with body fluids.

10. **Ask and assist resident to participate in washing.**
    Promotes independence.

11. **Uncover only one part of the body at a time. Place a towel under the body part being washed.**
    Promotes resident's dignity and right to privacy. Also helps keep resident warm.

12. **Wash, rinse, and dry one part of the body at a time. Start at the head, working down, and completing front first.**

    Eyes and Face: **Wash face with wet washcloth (no soap) beginning with the eyes, using a different area of the washcloth for each eye, washing inner aspect to outer aspect. Wash the face from the middle outward using firm but gentle strokes (Fig. 5-3). Wash the neck and ears and behind the ears. Rinse and pat dry.**

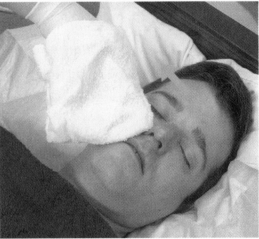

Fig. 5-3.

Arms: **Wash arm and underarm. Use long strokes from the shoulder down to the elbow. Rinse and pat dry. Wash the elbow. Wash, rinse, and dry from the elbow down to the wrist (Fig. 5-4).**

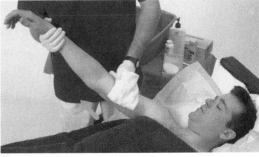

Fig. 5-4.

Wash the hand in a basin. Provide nail care (see procedure later in this chapter) only if it has been assigned.

Personal Care Skills

Chest and Abdomen: Wash, rinse, and pat dry both, only uncovering one part at a time. For a female resident: wash, rinse, and dry breasts and under breasts.

Legs: Wash the thigh. Use long downward strokes. Rinse and pat dry. Do the same from the knee to the ankle (Fig. 5-5).

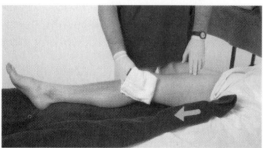

Fig. 5-5.

Wash the foot and between the toes in a basin (Fig. 5-6). Rinse foot and pat dry. Provide nail care (see procedure later in this chapter) only if it has been assigned.

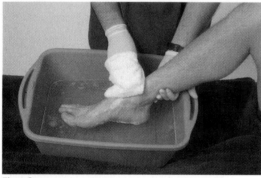

Fig. 5-6.

Back: Help resident move to the center of the bed, then turn onto his side so his or her back is facing you. Wash the back, neck, and buttocks with long, downward strokes. Rinse and pat dry (Fig. 5-7).

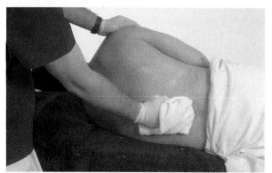

Fig. 5-7.

13. Put on gloves (if you haven't already done so) before washing perineal area.

14. Change bath water. Wash, rinse, and dry perineal area, working from front to back.

For a female resident: Wash the perineum with soap and water from *front to back*, using single strokes (Fig. 5-8).

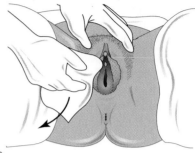

Fig. 5-8.

Do not wash from the back to the front, as this may cause infection. Use a clean area of washcloth or clean washcloth for each stroke. First wipe the center of the perineum, then each side. Then spread the labia majora, the outside folds of perineal skin that protect the urinary meatus and the vaginal opening. Wipe from front to back on each side. Rinse the area in the same way. Dry entire perineal area moving from front to back, using a blotting motion with towel. Ask resident to turn on her side. Wash, rinse, and dry buttocks and anal area. Cleanse the anal area without contaminating the perineal area.

For a male resident: If the resident is uncircumcised, retract the foreskin first. Gently push skin towards the base of penis.

Hold the penis by the shaft and wash in a circular motion from the tip down to the base. Use a clean area of washcloth or clean washcloth for each stroke (Fig. 5-9).

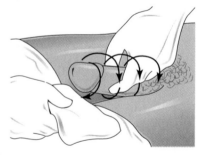

Fig. 5-9.

Rinse the penis. Then wash the scrotum and groin. The groin is the area from the pubis to the upper thighs. Rinse and pat dry. If resident is uncircumcised, gently return foreskin to normal position. Ask the resident to turn on his side. Wash, rinse, and dry buttocks and anal area. Cleanse the anal area without contaminating the perineal area.

15. **Apply lotion and deodorant. Do not apply lotion between the toes.**
Moisture between toes can promote fungus growth.

16. **Remove and dispose of gloves properly.**

17. **Put clean gown on resident. Assist resident to a position of safety and comfort and replace bedding.**

18. **Return bed to appropriate level. Put signaling device within resident's reach.**
Lowering the bed provides for safety. Signaling device allows resident to communicate with staff as necessary.

19. **Place soiled clothing and linens in appropriate containers.**

20. **Empty, rinse, and wipe bath basin and return to proper storage.**

21. **Wash hands.**
Provides for infection control.

22. **Report any changes in resident to the nurse.**
Provides nurse with information to assess resident.

23. **Document procedure according to facility guidelines.**
What you write is a legal record of what you did. If you don't document it, legally it didn't happen.

A partial bath is done on days when a complete bed bath or shower is not done. It includes washing the face, underarms, and hands, and performing perineal care.

Shampooing in bed

Equipment: shampoo, hair conditioner if requested, 2 bath towels, washcloth, bath thermometer, pitcher or hand-held shower or sink attachment, waterproof pad, bath blanket, trough, basin, comb and brush, hair dryer

1. **Wash hands.**
Provides for infection control.

2. **Identify yourself to resident by name. Address resident by name.**
Resident has right to know identity of his or her caregiver. Addressing resident by name shows respect and establishes correct identification.

3. **Explain procedure to resident, speaking clearly, slowly, and directly, maintaining face-to-face contact whenever possible.**
Promotes understanding and independence.

4. **Provide for resident's privacy during procedure with curtain, screen, or door.**
Maintains resident's right to privacy and dignity.

5. **Adjust bed to a safe working level, usually waist high. Remove pillow.**
Prevents injury to you and to resident.

6. **Test water temperature with thermometer or your wrist. Ensure it is safe. Water temperature should be 105° F. Have resident check water temperature. Adjust if necessary.**
Resident's sense of touch may be different than yours; therefore, resident is best able to identify a comfortable water temperature.

7. **Raise the side rail farthest from you.**

8. **Place the waterproof pad underneath the resident's head and shoulders.**
Protects bed linen.

9. **Place collection container under resident's head (e.g., trough, basin). Place one towel across the resident's shoulders.**

10. **Protect resident's eyes with dry washcloth.**

11. **Wet hair and apply shampoo.**

12. **Lather and massage scalp with fingertips (Fig. 5-10). Do not scratch the scalp.**

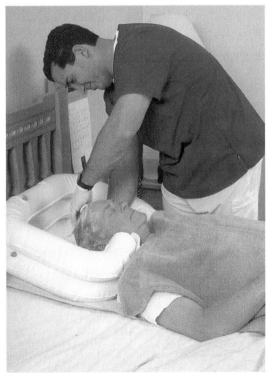

Fig. 5-10.

13. **Rinse hair until water runs clear. Apply conditioner and rinse as directed on container.**

14. **Cover resident's hair with clean towel. Dry his face with washcloth used to protect eyes.**

15. **Remove trough and waterproof covering.**

16. Raise head of bed.

17. Gently rub the scalp and hair with the towel.

18. Dry and comb resident's hair according to resident preference. (See procedure later in the chapter.)

19. Return bed to appropriate level.
    Lowering the bed provides for safety.

20. Before leaving resident, place signaling device within resident's reach.
    Allows resident to communicate with staff as necessary.

21. Empty, rinse, and wipe bath basin/pitcher and return to proper storage.

22. Clean comb/brush and return hairdryer and comb/brush to proper storage.

23. Place soiled linen in soiled linen container.

24. Wash hands.
    Provides for infection control.

25. Report any changes in resident to nurse.
    Provides nurse with information to assess resident.

26. Document procedure according to facility guidelines.
    What you write is a legal record of what you did. If you don't document it, legally it didn't happen.

Many people prefer showers or tub baths to bed baths (Fig. 5-11 and Fig. 5-12). Check with the nurse first to make sure a shower or tub bath is appropriate.

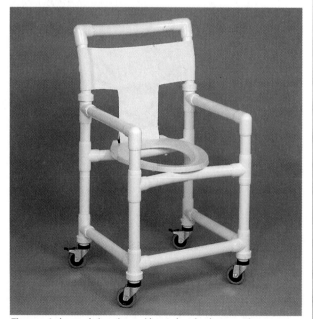

Fig. 5-11. A shower chair assists residents who take showers. (Photo courtesy of Innovative Products Unlimited)

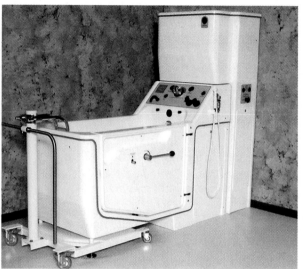

Fig. 5-12. A common style of tub in nursing homes. (Photo courtesy of Lee Penner of Penner Tubs)

GUIDELINES
Safety for Showers and Tub Baths

- Clean tub or shower before and after use.

- Make sure bathroom or shower room floor is dry.

- Be familiar with available safety and assistive devices. Check that hand rails, grab bars, and lifts are in working order.

- Have resident use safety bars when getting into or out of the tub or shower.

- Some facilities undress residents in their rooms before transporting them to the shower room. If so, cover resident while transporting to and from shower or tub room. It provides warmth and privacy. Other facilities transport residents to the shower room and undress them there.

- Place all needed items within reach.

- Do not leave resident alone.

- Avoid using bath oils. They make surfaces slippery.

- Test water temperature with thermometer or your wrist before resident gets into shower. Water temperature should be no more than 105° F. Make sure temperature is comfortable for resident.

RR *Privacy is very important when transporting residents to the shower room and during the shower. Make sure the body is not unnecessarily exposed.*

Giving a shower

Equipment: bath blanket, soap, shampoo, bath thermometer, 2-4 washcloths, 2-4 bath towels, clean gown and robe or clothes, gloves, lotion, deodorant

1. **Wash hands.**

   Provides for infection control.

2. **Identify yourself to resident by name. Address resident by name.**

   Resident has right to know identity of his or her caregiver. Addressing resident by name shows respect and establishes correct identification.

3. **Explain procedure to resident, speaking clearly, slowly, and directly, maintaining face-to-face contact whenever possible.**

   Promotes understanding and independence.

4. **Provide for resident's privacy during procedure with curtain, screen, or door.**

   Maintains resident's right to privacy and dignity.

5. **Clean shower area and shower chair.**

   Reduces pathogens and prevents the spread of infection.

6. **If using a shower chair, place it into position and lock wheels. Safely transfer resident into shower chair.**

   Chair may slide if resident attempts to get up.

7. **Turn on water. Test water temperature with thermometer. Water temperature should be no more than 105° F. Have resident check water temperature.**

   Resident's sense of touch may be different than yours; therefore, resident is best able to identify a comfortable water temperature.

8. **Put on gloves.**

   Protects you from coming into contact with body fluids.

9. **Help resident remove clothing. Drape resident with bath blanket.**

   Maintains resident's dignity and right to privacy by not exposing body. Keeps resident warm.

10. **Stay with resident during procedure.**

    Provides for resident's safety.

11. **Push shower chair into shower.**

12. **Let resident wash as much as possible. Assist to wash the face.**

    Encourages resident to be independent.

13. **Help resident shampoo and rinse hair.**

14. **Assist to wash and rinse the entire body, moving from head to toe.**

15. **Turn off water. Roll resident out of shower.**

16. **Give resident towel(s) and assist to pat dry. Remember to pat dry under the breasts, between skin folds, in the perineal area, and between toes.**

    Patting dry prevents skin tears and reduces chafing.

17. **Place soiled clothing and linens in appropriate containers.**

18. **Apply lotion and deodorant.**

19. **Remove gloves and wash hands.**

    Provides for infection control.

20. **Help resident dress and comb hair and return to room.**

    Combing hair in shower room allows resident to maintain dignity when returning to room.

21. **Before leaving resident, place signaling device within resident's reach.**

    Allows resident to communicate with staff as necessary.

22. **Report any changes in resident to nurse.**

    Provides nurse with information to assess resident.

23. **Document procedure according to facility guidelines.**

    What you write is a legal record of what you did. If you don't document it, legally it didn't happen.

Information on giving a back rub is later in the chapter, in the section on skin care.

Unit 3: Describe guidelines for assisting with grooming

When assisting with grooming, always allow residents to do all they can for themselves. Let them make as many choices as possible. Follow the instructions in the care plan for what care to provide. Some residents may have particular ways of grooming themselves, or they may have routines. These routines remain important even when people are elderly, sick, or disabled (Fig. 5-13). Remember, some residents may be embarrassed or depressed because they need help with grooming tasks they performed for themselves most their lives. Be sensitive to this.

Personal Care Skills

Personal Care Skills

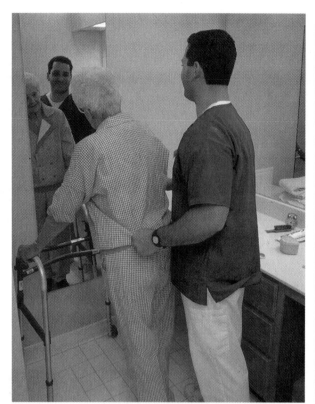
Fig. 5-13. Being well-groomed helps people feel good about themselves.

Nail care should only be provided if it has specifically been assigned. Never cut a resident's toenails. Poor circulation can lead to infection if skin is accidentally cut while caring for nails. In a diabetic resident, such an infection can lead to a severe wound or even amputation. (See chapter 8 for more information on diabetes.)

If you are directed to provide nail care for a resident, be sure you know exactly what care you are assigned to provide.

Providing fingernail care

Equipment: orangewood stick, emery board, lotion, basin, soap, washcloth, 2 towels, bath thermometer

1. **Wash hands.**

   Provides for infection control.

2. **Identify yourself to resident by name. Address resident by name.**

   Resident has right to know identity of his or her caregiver. Addressing resident by name shows respect and establishes correct identification.

3. **Explain procedure to resident, speaking clearly, slowly, and directly, maintaining**

face-to-face contact whenever possible.

Promotes understanding and independence.

4. **Provide for resident's privacy during procedure with curtain, screen, or door.**

   Maintains resident's right to privacy and dignity.

5. **Adjust bed to a safe working level, usually waist high, if in bed.**

   Prevents injury to you and to resident.

6. **Test water temperature with thermometer or your wrist and ensure it is safe. Water temperature should be 105° F. Have resident check water temperature. Adjust if necessary.**

   Resident's sense of touch may be different than yours; therefore, resident is best able to identify a comfortable water temperature.

7. **Immerse resident's hands in basin of water, which is placed at a comfortable level for the resident. Soak hands for two to four minutes.**

   Nail care is easier if nails are first softened.

8. **Remove hands. Wash hands with soapy washcloth. Rinse. Pat hands dry with towel, including between fingers.**

9. **Clean under nails with orangewood stick (Fig. 5-14).**

   Most pathogens on hands come from beneath the nails.

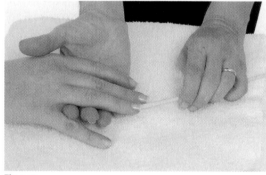
Fig. 5-14.

10. **Wipe orangewood stick on towel after each nail.**

11. **Groom nails with file or emery board. File in a curve.**

    Filing in a curve smoothes nails and eliminates edges, which may catch on clothes or tear skin.

12. **Finish with nails smooth and free of rough edges.**

13. **Apply lotion from fingertips to wrist.**

14. **Return bed to appropriate level if previously adjusted.**

    Lowering the bed provides for safety.

15. **Before leaving resident, place signaling device within resident's reach.**
Allows resident to communicate with staff as necessary.

16. **Empty, rinse, and wipe basin, and return to proper storage.**

17. **Dispose of soiled linen in the soiled linen container.**

18. **Wash hands.**
Provides for infection control.

19. **Report any changes in resident to the nurse.**
Provides nurse with information to assess resident.

20. **Document procedure according to facility guidelines.**
What you write is a legal record of what you did. If you don't document it, legally it didn't happen.

Never use the same nail equipment on more than one resident.

Providing foot care

Equipment: basin, bath mat, soap, lotion, washcloth, 2 towels, bath thermometer, clean socks

Support the foot and ankle throughout procedure.

1. **Wash hands.**
Provides for infection control.

2. **Identify yourself to resident by name. Address resident by name.**
Resident has right to know identity of his or her caregiver. Addressing resident by name shows respect and establishes correct identification.

3. **Explain procedure to resident, speaking clearly, slowly, and directly, maintaining face-to-face contact whenever possible.**
Promotes understanding and independence.

4. **Provide for resident's privacy during procedure with curtain, screen, or door.**
Maintains resident's right to privacy and dignity.

5. **Adjust bed to a safe working level, usually waist high, if in bed.**
Prevents injury to you and to resident.

6. **Test water temperature with thermometer or your wrist and ensure it is safe. Water temperature should be 105° F. Have resident check water temperature. Adjust if necessary.**
Resident's sense of touch may be different than yours; therefore, resident is best able to identify a comfortable water temperature.

7. **Place basin on the bath mat.**

8. **Remove socks. Completely submerge feet in water. Soak the feet for five to ten minutes.**

9. **Remove one foot from water. Wash entire foot, including between the toes and around nail beds, with soapy washcloth (Fig. 5-15).**

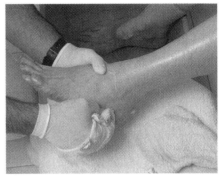

Fig. 5-15.

10. **Rinse entire foot, including between the toes.**

11. **Dry entire foot, including between the toes.**

12. **Repeat steps 8 through 10 for the other foot.**

13. **Put lotion in hand. Warm lotion by rubbing hands together.**

14. **Massage lotion into entire foot (top and bottom), removing excess (if any) with a towel.**

15. **Assist resident to replace socks.**

16. **Return bed to appropriate level if previously adjusted.**
Lowering the bed provides for safety.

17. **Before leaving resident, place signaling device within resident's reach.**
Allows resident to communicate with staff as necessary.

18. **Empty, rinse, and wipe basin, and return to proper storage.**

19. **Dispose of soiled linen in the soiled linen container.**

20. **Wash hands.**
Provides for infection control.

21. **Report any changes in resident to the nurse.**
Provides nurse with information to assess resident.

22. **Document procedure according to facility guidelines.**
What you write is a legal record of what you did. If you don't document it, legally it didn't happen.

Combing or brushing hair

Equipment: comb, brush, towel, mirror, hair care items requested by resident

Personal Care Skills

Use hair care products that the resident prefers for his or her type of hair.

1. **Wash hands.**

   Provides for infection control.

2. **Identify yourself to resident by name. Address resident by name.**

   Resident has right to know identity of his or her caregiver. Addressing resident by name shows respect and establishes correct identification.

3. **Explain procedure to resident, speaking clearly, slowly, and directly, maintaining face-to-face contact whenever possible.**

   Promotes understanding and independence.

4. **Provide for resident's privacy during procedure with curtain, screen, or door.**

   Maintains resident's right to privacy and dignity.

5. **Raise head of bed so resident is sitting up. Place a towel under the head or around the shoulders.**

   Puts resident in more natural position.

6. **Remove any hair pins, hair ties and clips.**

7. **Remove tangles first by dividing hair into small sections. Gently comb out from ends of hair to scalp.**

   Reduces hair breakage, scalp pain and irritation.

8. **After tangles are removed, brush two-inch sections of hair at a time. Brush from roots to ends (Fig. 5-16).**

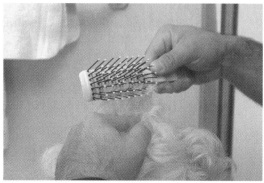

Fig. 5-16.

9. **Style hair in the way resident prefers. Avoid childish hairstyles. Each resident may prefer different styles and different hair products. Offer mirror to resident.**

   Each resident has right to choose. Promotes resident's independence.

10. **Return bed to appropriate level.**

    Provides for safety.

11. **Before leaving resident, place signaling device within resident's reach.**

    Allows resident to communicate with staff as necessary.

12. **Return supplies to proper storage. Clean hair from brush/comb.**

13. **Dispose of soiled linen in the soiled linen container.**

14. **Wash hands.**

    Provides for infection control.

15. **Report any changes in resident to nurse.**

    Provides nurse with information to assess resident.

16. **Document procedure according to facility guidelines.**

    What you write is a legal record of what you did. If you don't document it, legally it didn't happen.

Shaving a resident

Be sure the resident wants you to shave him or help him shave before you begin. Check with the nurse to know which type of razor the resident uses.

A **safety razor** has a sharp blade, but with a special safety casing to help prevent cuts. This type of razor requires shaving cream or soap.

An **electric razor** is the safest and easiest type of razor to use. It does not require soap or shaving cream.

A **disposable razor** requires shaving cream or soap. It is discarded after use.

Equipment: basin, 2 towels, washcloth, bath thermometer, mirror, shaving cream or soap, after-shave (for male residents), gloves, razor

1. **Wash hands.**

   Provides for infection control.

2. **Identify yourself to resident by name. Address resident by name.**

   Resident has right to know identity of his or her caregiver. Addressing resident by name shows respect and establishes correct identification.

3. **Explain procedure to resident, speaking clearly, slowly, and directly, maintaining face-to-face contact whenever possible.**

   Promotes understanding and independence.

4. **Provide for resident's privacy during procedure with curtain, screen, or door.**

   Maintains resident's right to privacy and dignity.

5. **Raise head of bed so resident is sitting up.**

   Puts resident in more natural position.

Shaving using a safety razor:

6. **Fill bath basin halfway with warm water.**

   Hot water opens pores and causes irritation.

7. **Drape towel under resident's chin.**
   Protects resident's clothing and bed linen.

8. **Apply gloves.**
   Shaving may cause bleeding. Promotes infection control.

9. **Moisten beard with warm washcloth. Put shaving cream or soap over area.**
   Softens skin and hair.

10. **Hold skin taut and shave beard in downward strokes on face and upward strokes on neck. Rinse razor often in warm water to keep it clean and wet (Fig. 5-17).**
    Maximizes hair removal by shaving in the direction of hair growth.

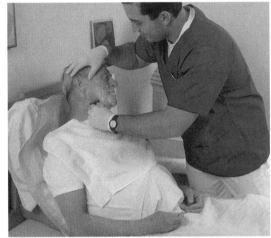
Fig. 5-17.

11. **Offer mirror to resident.**
    Promotes independence.

12. **Wash, rinse, and dry face after the shave. Apply after-shave lotion as requested.**
    Removes soap, which may cause irritation. Improves resident's self-esteem

13. **Remove towel.**

14. **Remove gloves.**

Shaving using an electric razor:

6. **Do not use an electric razor near any water source, when oxygen is in use, or if resident has a pacemaker.**
   Electricity near water may cause electrocution. Electricity near oxygen may cause an explosion. Electricity near some pacemakers may cause an irregular heartbeat.

7. **Drape towel under resident's chin.**
   Protects resident's clothing and bed linen.

8. **Apply gloves.**
   Shaving may cause bleeding.

9. **Apply pre-shave lotion as resident wishes.**

10. **Hold skin taut. Shave with smooth, even movements (Fig. 5-18).**
    Smoothes out skin. Shave beard with back and forth motion in direction of beard growth with foil shaver. Shave beard in circular motion with three-head shaver.

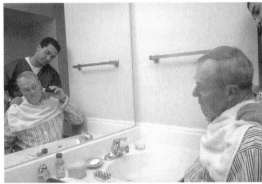
Fig. 5-18.

11. **Offer mirror to resident.**
    Promotes independence.

12. **Apply after-shave lotion as resident wishes.**
    Improves resident's self-esteem.

13. **Remove towel.**

14. **Remove gloves.**

Final steps:

15. **Make sure that resident and environment are free of loose hairs.**

16. **Return bed to appropriate level.**
    Provides for safety.

17. **Before leaving resident, place signaling device within resident's reach.**
    Allows resident to communicate with staff as necessary.

18. ***For safety razor*: Rinse safety razor. *For disposable razor*: Dispose of a disposable razor in appropriate biohazard container. *For electric razor*: Clean head of electric razor. Remove whiskers from razor. Re-cap shaving head. Return razor to case.**

19. **Return supplies and equipment to proper storage.**

20. **Wash hands.**
    Provides for infection control.

21. **Report any changes in resident to the nurse.**
    Provides nurse with information to assess resident.

22. **Document procedure according to facility guidelines.**
    What you write is a legal record of what you did. If you don't document it, legally it didn't happen.

Personal Care Skills

Unit 4: Identify guidelines for good oral hygiene

Oral care, or care of the mouth, teeth, and gums, is performed at least twice each day. Oral care should be done after breakfast and after the last meal or snack of the day. It may also be done before a resident eats. Oral care includes brushing teeth and tongue, flossing teeth, and caring for dentures (Fig. 5-19).

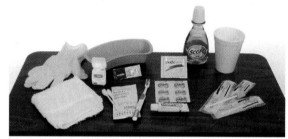

Fig. 5-19. Some supplies needed for oral care.

When you provide oral care, observe the resident's mouth.

OBSERVING AND REPORTING
Oral Care

- irritation
- infection
- raised areas
- coated tongue
- ulcers, such as canker sores or small, painful, white sores
- flaky, white spots
- dry and cracked or chapped lips
- loose or decayed teeth
- swollen, bleeding, or whitish gums
- breath that smells bad or fruity

Providing mouth care

Equipment: toothbrush, toothpaste, emesis basin, gloves, towel, glass of water

1. **Wash hands.**
   Provides for infection control.

2. **Identify yourself to resident by name. Address resident by name.**
   Resident has right to know identity of his or her caregiver. Addressing resident by name shows respect and establishes correct identification.

3. **Explain procedure to resident, speaking clearly, slowly, and directly, maintaining face-to-face contact whenever possible.**
   Promotes understanding and independence.

4. **Provide for resident's privacy during procedure with curtain, screen, or door.**
   Maintains resident's right to privacy and dignity.

5. **Adjust bed to a safe working level, usually waist high. Make sure resident is in an upright sitting position.**
   Prevents injury to you and to resident. Prevents fluids from running down resident's throat, causing choking.

6. **Put on gloves.**
   Brushing may cause gums to bleed.

7. **Place towel across resident's chest.**
   Protects resident's clothing and bed linen.

8. **Wet brush and put on small amount of toothpaste.**
   Water helps distribute toothpaste.

9. **Clean entire mouth (including tongue and all surfaces of teeth), using gentle motions. First brush upper teeth, then lower teeth. Use short strokes and brush back and forth.**
   Brushing upper teeth first minimizes production of saliva in lower part of mouth.

10. **Hold emesis basin to the resident's chin (Fig. 5-20).**

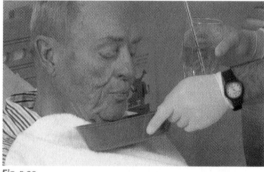

Fig. 5-20.

11. **Have resident rinse mouth with water and spit into emesis basin.**
    Removes food particles and toothpaste.

12. **Wipe resident's mouth and remove towel.**

13. **Dispose of soiled linen in the soiled linen container.**

14. **Clean and return supplies to proper storage.**

15. **Remove gloves. Dispose of gloves properly.**

16. **Return bed to appropriate level.**
Lowering the bed provides for safety.

17. **Before leaving resident, place signaling device within resident's reach.**
Allows resident to communicate with staff as necessary.

18. **Wash hands.**
Provides for infection control.

19. **Report any problems with teeth, mouth, tongue, and lips to nurse. This includes odor, cracking, sores, bleeding, and any discoloration.**
Provides nurse with information to assess resident.

20. **Document procedure according to facility guidelines.**
What you write is a legal record of what you did. If you don't document it, legally it didn't happen.

👁 *You must brush the tongue when providing oral care.*

Flossing the teeth removes plaque and tartar buildup around the gum line and between the teeth. Teeth may be flossed immediately after or before they are brushed, as the resident prefers.

Flossing teeth

Equipment: floss, cup with water, emesis basin, gloves, towel

1. **Wash hands.**
Provides for infection control.

2. **Identify yourself to resident by name. Address resident by name.**
Resident has right to know identity of his or her caregiver. Addressing resident by name shows respect and establishes correct identification.

3. **Explain procedure to resident, speaking clearly, slowly, and directly, maintaining face-to-face contact whenever possible.**
Promotes understanding and independence.

4. **Provide for resident's privacy during procedure with curtain, screen, or door.**
Maintains resident's right to privacy and dignity.

5. **Adjust the bed to a safe working level. Make sure the resident is in an upright sitting position.**
Prevents injury to you and to resident. Prevents fluids from running down resident's throat, causing choking.

6. **Put on gloves.**
Flossing may cause gums to bleed.

7. **Wrap the ends of floss securely around each index finger (Fig. 5-21).**

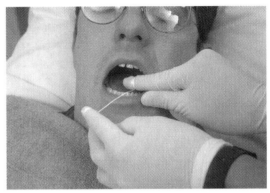

Fig. 5-21.

8. **Starting with the back teeth, place floss between teeth and move it down the surface of the tooth using a gentle sawing motion (Fig. 5-22).**
Being gentle protects gums.

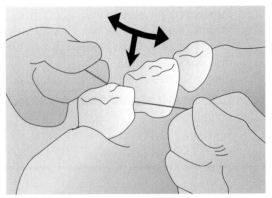

Fig. 5-22.

Continue to the gum line. At the gum line, curve the floss into a letter C, slip it gently into the space between the gum and tooth, then go back up, scraping that side of the tooth (Fig. 5-23).

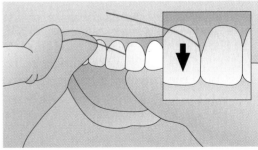

Fig. 5-23.

Repeat this on the side of the other tooth.
Removes food and prevents tooth decay.

9. **After every two or three teeth, unwind floss**

from your fingers and move it so you are using a clean area. Floss all teeth.

10. **Offer water to rinse debris from the mouth into the basin.**
    Flossing loosens food. Rinsing removes it.

11. **Offer resident a face towel when done flossing all teeth.**
    Promotes dignity.

12. **Dispose of soiled linen in the soiled linen container.**

13. **Clean and return supplies to proper storage.**

14. **Remove and dispose of gloves properly.**

15. **Return bed to appropriate level.**
    Lowering the bed provides for safety.

16. **Before leaving resident, place signaling device within resident's reach.**
    Allows resident to communicate with staff as necessary.

17. **Wash hands.**
    Provides for infection control.

18. **Report any problems with teeth, mouth, tongue, and lips to nurse. This includes odor, cracking, sores, bleeding, and any discoloration.**
    Provides nurse with information to assess resident.

19. **Document procedure according to facility guidelines.**
    What you write is a legal record of what you did. If you don't document it, legally it didn't happen.

Dentures are artificial teeth. They are expensive to replace. Take good care of them. Handle dentures carefully to avoid breaking or chipping them. Notify the nurse if a resident's dentures do not fit properly, are chipped, or are missing.

Cleaning and storing dentures

Equipment: denture brush or toothbrush, denture cleanser or toothpaste, labeled denture cup, 2 towels, gloves

1. **Wash hands.**
   Provides for infection control.

2. **Put on gloves.**
   Prevents you from coming into contact with body fluids.

3. **Line sink/basin with a towel(s).**
   Prevents dentures from breaking if dropped.

4. **Rinse dentures in cool running water before brushing them. Do not use hot water.**
   Hot water may damage dentures.

5. **Apply toothpaste or cleanser to toothbrush.**

6. **Brush dentures on all surfaces (Fig. 5-24).**

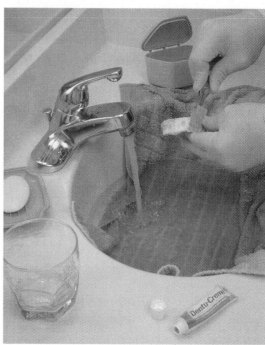

Fig. 5-24.

7. **Rinse all surfaces of dentures under cool running water. Do not use hot water.**
   Hot water may damage dentures.

8. **Rinse denture cup before placing clean dentures in it.**
   Removes pathogens.

9. **Place dentures in clean denture cup with solution or cool water (Fig. 5-25). Make sure cup is labeled with resident's name.**

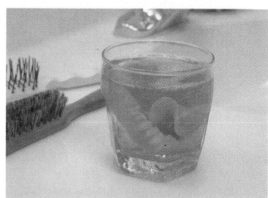

Fig. 5-25.

10. **Clean and return the equipment to proper storage.**

11. **Dispose of towels in appropriate container.**

12. **Remove your gloves. Dispose of gloves properly.**

13. **Wash hands.**
    Provides for infection control.

14. **Report any changes in appearance of dentures to the nurse.**
    Provides nurse with information to assess resident.

15. **Document procedure according to facility guidelines.**
    What you write is a legal record of what you did. If you don't document it, legally it didn't happen.

Although residents who are unconscious cannot eat, breathing through the mouth causes saliva to dry in the mouth. Good mouth care needs to be performed more frequently to keep the mouth clean and moist. Swabs with a mixture of lemon juice and glycerine are sometimes used to soothe the gums. But these may further dry the gums if used too often. Follow the care plan regarding the use of swabs.

With unconscious residents, it is important to use as little liquid as possible when performing mouth care. Because the person's swallowing reflex is weak, he or she is at risk for aspiration. **Aspiration** is the inhalation of food or drink into the lungs. Aspiration can cause pneumonia or death. Chapter 7 has more information on aspiration.

Providing mouth care for the unconscious resident

Equipment: sponge swabs, padded tongue blade, towel, emesis basin, gloves, lip moisturizer, cleaning solution (check the care plan)

1. **Wash hands.**
   Provides for infection control.

2. **Identify self to resident by name. Identify and address resident by name. Even residents who are unconscious may be able to hear you. Always speak to them as you would to any resident.**
   Resident has right to know identity of his or her caregiver. Addressing resident by name shows respect and establishes correct identification.

3. **Explain procedure to resident, speaking clearly, slowly, and directly, maintaining face-to-face contact whenever possible.**
   Promotes understanding and independence.

4. **Provide for resident's privacy throughout procedure with curtain, screen, or door.**
   Maintains resident's right to privacy and dignity.

5. **Adjust bed to a safe working level, usually waist high.**
   Prevents injury to you and to resident.

6. **Put on gloves.**
   Protects you from coming into contact with body fluids.

7. **Turn resident's head to the side and place a towel under his cheek and chin. Place an emesis basin next to the cheek and chin for excess fluid.**
   Protects resident's clothing and bed linen.

8. **Hold mouth open with padded tongue blade.**
   Enables you to safely clean mouth.

9. **Dip swab in cleaning solution. Wipe teeth, gums, tongue, and inside surfaces of mouth, changing swab frequently. Repeat until the mouth is clean (Fig. 5-26).**
   Stimulates gums and removes mucus.

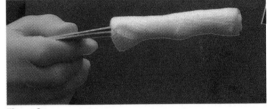

Fig. 5-26.

10. **Rinse with clean swab dipped in water.**
    Removes solution from mouth.

11. **Remove the towel and basin. Pat lips or face dry if needed. Apply lip moisturizer.**
    Prevents lips from drying and cracking. Improves resident's comfort.

12. **Dispose of soiled linen in the soiled linen container.**

13. **Clean and return supplies to proper storage.**

14. **Remove your gloves. Dispose of gloves properly.**

15. **Return bed to appropriate level.**
    Lowering the bed provides for safety.

16. **Before leaving resident, place signaling device within resident's reach.**
    Allows resident to communicate with staff as necessary.

Personal Care Skills

17. **Wash hands.**

    Provides for infection control.

18. **Report any changes in resident to the nurse.**

    Provides nurse with information to assess resident.

19. **Document procedure according to facility guidelines.**

    What you write is a legal record of what you did. If you don't document it, legally it didn't happen.

Unit 5: **List guidelines for assisting with dressing**

When assisting a resident with dressing, know what limitations he or she has. If he or she has a weakened side from a stroke or injury, that side is called the **affected** side. It will be weaker. Never refer to the weaker side as the "bad side," or talk about the "bad" leg or arm. Use the terms **weaker** or **involved** to refer to the affected side. The weaker arm is usually placed through a sleeve first (Fig. 5-27). When a leg is weak, it is easier if the resident sits down to pull the pants over both legs.

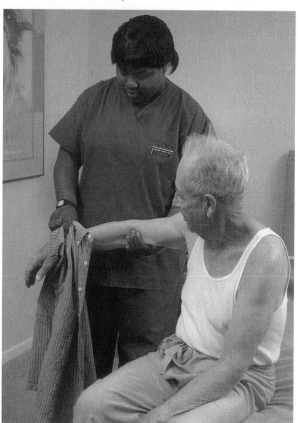

Fig. 5-27. When dressing, assist with the weaker side first.

Residents should do as much for themselves as they can when dressing. This includes choosing the clothes they will wear. This encourages independence and promotes self-care.

GUIDELINES
Helping a Resident Dress and Undress

- The resident's preferences should be asked and followed.

- Allow the resident to choose clothing for the day. However, check to see if it is clean, appropriate for the weather, and in good condition.

- Encourage the resident to dress in regular clothes rather than nightclothes.

- The resident should do as much to dress or undress himself as possible.

- Provide privacy.

- Front-fastening bras are easier for residents to manage by themselves.

- Place the weak arm or leg through the garment first, then the strong arm. When undressing, do the opposite.

Dressing a resident with an affected right arm

Equipment: clean clothes of resident's choice, non-skid footwear

1. **Wash hands.**

   Provides for infection control.

2. **Identify yourself to resident by name. Address resident by name.**

   Resident has right to know identity of his or her caregiver. Addressing resident by name shows respect and establishes correct identification.

3. **Explain procedure to resident, speaking clearly, slowly, and directly, maintaining face-to-face contact whenever possible.**

   Promotes understanding and independence.

4. **Provide for resident's privacy during procedure with curtain, screen, or door.**

   Maintains resident's right to privacy and dignity.

5. **Ask resident which outfit she would like to wear. Dress her in outfit of choice (Fig 5-28).**

   Promotes resident's right to choose.

6. **Remove resident's gown without completely exposing resident. Take off stronger side first when undressing.**
   Maintains resident's dignity and right to privacy by not exposing body.

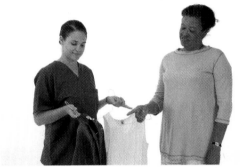

Fig. 5-28.

7. **Assist resident to put the right (affected) arm through the right sleeve of the shirt, sweater, or slip before placing garment on left (unaffected) arm.**
   Dressing affected side first requires less movement and reduces stress to joints.

8. **Assist resident to put on skirt, pants, or dress.**

9. **Place bed at a safe and appropriate level for resident, usually the lowest position.**

10. **Apply non-skid footwear.**
    Promotes resident's safety.

11. **Put on all items, moving resident's body gently and naturally, avoiding force and over-extension of limbs and joints.**
    Prevents injury to resident.

12. **Finish with resident dressed appropriately. Make sure clothing is right-side-out and zippers/buttons are fastened.**

13. **Place gown in soiled linen container.**

14. **Before leaving resident, place signaling device within resident's reach.**
    Allows resident to communicate with staff as necessary.

15. **Wash hands.**
    Provides for infection control.

16. **Report any changes in resident to the nurse.**
    Provides nurse with information to assess resident.

17. **Document procedure according to facility guidelines.**
    What you write is a legal record of what you did. If you don't document it, legally it didn't happen.

👁 *Always dress a resident's weaker or affected side first.*

IV stands for **intravenous**, or into a vein. Medication, nutrition, or fluids drip from a bag suspended on a pole through a tube and into the vein. Chapter 6 has more information on IVs.

GUIDELINES
Dressing a Resident with an IV

Dressing and undressing residents with IVs requires special care.

- Remove or assist in removing clothing from the side without the IV. Then hold garment while undressing the side with the IV.

- Slide clothing over the tubing. Lift the IV bag off the hook and pull the gown over the bag (Fig. 5-29).

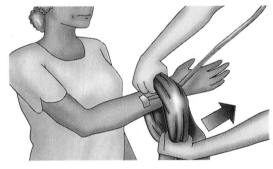

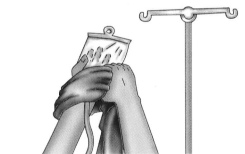

Fig. 5-29.

- Always keep bag above IV site on body.

- Apply clean clothing first to side with the IV. Slide the correct arm opening over the bag, then over the tubing and the resident's IV arm.

Unit 6: **Explain guidelines for assisting with toileting**

Residents who are unable to get out of bed to go to the bathroom may be given a bed-

Personal Care Skills

pan, a urinal, or a fracture pan. A **fracture pan** is a bedpan that is flatter than the regular bedpan. It is used for residents who cannot assist with raising their hips onto a regular bedpan (Fig. 5-30).

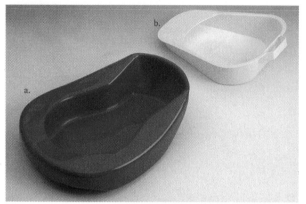

Fig. 5-30. a) Standard pan and b) fracture pan.

Women will use a bedpan for urination and bowel movements. Men will generally use a urinal for urination and a bedpan for a bowel movement (Fig. 5-31). This equipment should be rinsed with a facility-approved disinfectant after each use and kept in the bathroom between uses. Never place this equipment on an overbed or side table.

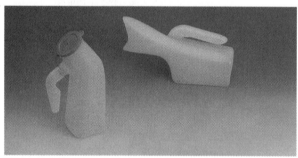

Fig. 5-31. Urinals.

Residents who are able to get out of bed but cannot walk to the bathroom may use a portable commode. A **portable commode** is a chair with a toilet seat and a removable container underneath (Fig. 5-32).

Wastes such as urine and feces can carry infection. Always dispose of wastes in the toilet. Be careful not to spill or splash. Wear gloves when handling bedpans, urinals, or basins that contain wastes, including dirty bath water. Wash these containers tho-

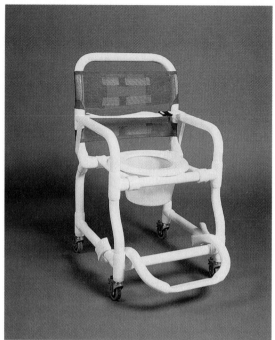

Fig. 5-32. A portable commode.

roughly with an approved disinfectant. Rinse and dry and return to storage.

Assisting resident with use of bedpan

Equipment: bedpan, bedpan cover, protective pad or sheet, toilet paper, washcloths or wipes, gloves

1. **Wash hands.**
   Provides for infection control.

2. **Identify yourself to resident by name. Address resident by name.**
   Resident has right to know identity of his or her caregiver. Addressing resident by name shows respect and establishes correct identification.

3. **Explain procedure to resident, speaking clearly, slowly, and directly, maintaining face-to-face contact whenever possible.**
   Promotes understanding and independence.

4. **Provide for resident's privacy during procedure with curtain, screen, or door.**
   Maintains resident's right to privacy and dignity.

5. **Apply gloves.**
   Prevents you from coming into contact with body fluids.

6. **Before placing bedpan, lower head of bed.**
   When bed is flat, resident can be moved without working against gravity.

7. **Place a protective pad under the resident's buttocks and hips.**
   Prevents linen from being soiled. Promotes infection control.

8. Ask resident to remove undergarments or help him do so.
   Promotes independence.

9. If resident is able, ask him to raise hips by pushing with feet and hands. Place bedpan correctly under resident's buttocks (Standard bedpan: Position bedpan so wider end of pan is aligned with resident's buttocks (Fig. 5-33); Fracture pan: Position bedpan with handle toward foot of bed).

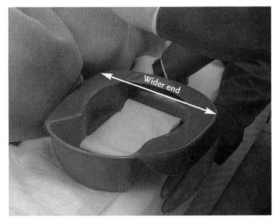

Fig. 5-33.

10. Raise head of bed after placing bedpan under resident.
    Puts resident in comfortable position for voiding.

11. Put toilet tissue within resident's reach.

12. Leave signaling device within resident's reach while resident is using bedpan. Ask resident to signal when finished.
    Ensures ability to communicate need for assistance.

13. Return and lower head of bed.
    Places resident in proper position to remove pan.

14. Remove bedpan carefully. Cover bedpan.
    Promotes infection control and odor control. Provides dignity for resident.

15. Provide perineal care if assistance is needed. Remember to wipe female residents from front to back.
    Prevents spread of pathogens, which may cause urinary tract infection.

16. Empty contents of bedpan into toilet. Note color, odor, and consistency of contents.
    Changes may be first sign of medical problem.

17. Rinse bedpan, pouring rinse water into toilet, and return to proper storage.

18. After storing bedpan, remove and dispose of gloves properly.

19. Assist resident to wash hands after using bedpan. Dispose of soiled washcloth or wipes in proper container. Help resident put on undergarment.
    Handwashing is the best way to prevent the spread of infection.

20. Return bed to appropriate level.
    Lowering the bed provides for resident's safety.

21. Before leaving resident, place signaling device within resident's reach.
    Allows resident to communicate with staff as necessary.

22. Wash hands.
    Provides for infection control.

23. Report any changes in resident to the nurse.
    Provides nurse with information to assess resident.

24. Document procedure according to facility guidelines.
    What you write is a legal record of what you did. If you don't document it, legally it didn't happen.

☞ *Remember to position a standard bedpan so that the wider end is aligned with a resident's buttocks. A fracture pan should be positioned with the handle toward the foot of the bed.*

Assisting a male resident with a urinal

Equipment: urinal, protective pad or sheet, washcloths or wipes, gloves

1. Wash hands.
   Provides for infection control.

2. Identify yourself to resident by name. Address resident by name.
   Resident has right to know identity of his or her caregiver. Addressing resident by name shows respect and establishes correct identification.

3. Explain procedure to resident, speaking clearly, slowly, and directly, maintaining face-to-face contact whenever possible.
   Promotes understanding and independence.

4. Provide for resident's privacy during procedure with curtain, screen, or door.
   Maintains resident's right to privacy and dignity.

5. Apply gloves.
   Prevents you from coming into contact with body fluids.

6. Place a protective pad under the resident's buttocks and hips.
   Prevents linen from being soiled.

7. Hand the urinal to the resident. If the resident is not able to help himself, place urinal

between his legs and position penis inside the urinal (Fig. 5-34). Replace bed covers.

Promotes independence, dignity and privacy.

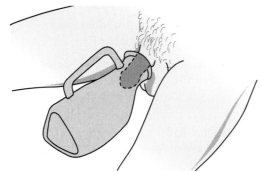

Fig. 5-34.

8. **Leave signaling device within resident's reach while resident is using urinal. Ask resident to signal when finished.**

Ensures ability to communicate need for assistance.

9. **Remove urinal; empty contents into toilet. Note color, odor, and qualities (e.g. cloudy) of contents.**

Changes may be first sign of medical problem.

10. **Rinse urinal, pouring rinse water into toilet, and return to proper storage.**

11. **After storing urinal, remove and dispose of gloves.**

12. **Assist resident to wash hands after using urinal. Dispose of soiled washcloth or wipes in proper container.**

Handwashing is the best way to prevent the spread of infection.

13. **Before leaving resident, place signaling device within resident's reach.**

Allows resident to communicate with staff as necessary.

14. **Wash hands.**

Provides for infection control.

15. **Report any changes in resident to the nurse.**

Provides nurse with information to assess resident.

16. **Document procedure according to facility guidelines.**

What you write is a legal record of what you did. If you don't document it, legally it didn't happen.

Helping a resident use a portable commode

Equipment: portable commode with basin, toilet paper, washcloths or wipes, gloves

1. **Wash hands.**

Provides for infection control.

2. **Identify yourself to resident by name.**

Address resident by name.

Resident has right to know identity of his or her caregiver. Addressing resident by name shows respect and establishes correct identification.

3. **Explain procedure to resident, speaking clearly, slowly, and directly, maintaining face-to-face contact whenever possible.**

Promotes understanding and independence.

4. **Provide for resident's privacy during procedure with curtain, screen, or door.**

Maintains resident's right to privacy and dignity.

5. **Help resident out of bed and to portable commode. Make sure resident is wearing non-skid shoes.**

6. **If needed, help resident remove clothing and sit comfortably on toilet seat. Put toilet tissue within resident's reach.**

7. **Leave signaling device within resident's reach while resident is using commode. Ask resident to signal when finished.**

Ensures ability to communicate need for assistance.

8. **Return and apply gloves.**

Prevents you from coming into contact with body fluids.

9. **Provide perineal care if assistance is needed. Remember to wipe female residents from front to back.**

Prevents spread of pathogens, which may cause urinary tract infection.

10. **Assist resident to wash hands after using commode. Dispose of soiled washcloth or wipes in proper container.**

Handwashing is the best way to prevent the spread of infection.

11. **Assist back to bed.**

12. **Remove waste container and empty contents into toilet. Note color, odor, and consistency of contents.**

Changes may be first sign of medical problem.

13. **Rinse container, pouring rinse water into toilet, and return to proper storage.**

14. **After storing container, remove and dispose of gloves properly.**

15. **Before leaving resident, place signaling device within resident's reach.**

Allows resident to communicate with staff as necessary.

16. **Wash hands.**

Provides for infection control.

17. **Report any changes in resident to the nurse.**

Provides nurse with information to assess resident.

Personal Care Skills

18. **Document procedure according to facility guidelines.**

    What you write is a legal record of what you did. If you don't document it, legally it didn't happen.

Some people cannot control the muscles of the bowels or bladder. They are said to be **incontinent**. Incontinence can occur in residents who are confined to bed, ill, paralyzed, or who have circulatory or nervous system diseases or injuries. Diarrhea can also cause temporary incontinence.

Residents who are incontinent need reassurance and understanding. Offer them a bedpan or take them to the bathroom more frequently. Keep them clean, dry, and free from odor. Some residents will wear disposable incontinence pads or briefs for adults. They should be changed often. Residents who are incontinent will need good skin care. Urine and feces are very irritating to the skin. They should be washed off completely by bathing and good perineal care.

📋 *The survey team will look to see that each resident's elimination needs are met. This includes a toileting schedule to lessen episodes of incontinence.*

Providing perineal care for an incontinent resident

Equipment: 2 clean protective pads, 4 washcloths or wipes, 1 towel, gloves, basin with warm water, soap, bath blanket, bath thermometer

1. **Wash hands.**

   Provides for infection control.

2. **Identify yourself to resident by name. Address resident by name.**

   Resident has right to know identity of his or her caregiver. Addressing resident by name shows respect and establishes correct identification.

3. **Explain procedure to resident, speaking clearly, slowly, and directly, maintaining face-to-face contact whenever possible.**

   Promotes understanding and independence.

4. **Provide for resident's privacy during proce-** dure with curtain, screen, or door.

   Maintains resident's right to privacy and dignity.

5. **Adjust bed to a safe working level, usually waist high.**

   Prevents injury to you and to resident.

6. **Lower head of bed. Position resident lying flat on his or her back. Raise the side rail farthest from you.**

7. **Test water temperature with thermometer or your wrist and ensure it is safe. Water temperature should be 105° to 109° F. Have resident check water temperature. Adjust if necessary.**

   Resident's sense of touch may be different than yours; therefore, resident is best able to identify a comfortable water temperature.

8. **Put on gloves.**

   Prevents you from coming into contact with body fluids.

9. **Remove soiled protective pad from underneath resident by turning resident on his side, away from you. (See procedure Turning a Resident later in this chapter.) Roll soiled pad into itself with wet side in/dry side out.**

   Keeps linen from getting wet.

10. **Place clean protective pad under his or her buttocks.**

    Keeps linen from getting wet.

11. **Return resident to lying on his back.**

12. **Cover resident with bath blanket.**

    Maintains resident's right to privacy and dignity.

13. **Expose perineal area only. Clean perineal area.**

    For a female resident: Wash the perineum with soap and water from *front to back*, using single strokes. Do not wash from the back to the front, as this may cause infection. Use a clean area of washcloth or clean washcloth for each stroke. First wipe the center of the perineum, then each side. Then spread the labia majora, the outside folds of perineal skin that protect the urinary meatus and the vaginal opening. Wipe from front to back on each side. Rinse the area in the same way. Dry entire perineal area moving from front to back, using a blotting motion with towel. Ask resident to turn on her side. Wash, rinse, and dry buttocks and anal area. Cleanse the anal area without contaminating the perineal area.

    For a male resident: If the resident is uncircumcised, retract the foreskin first. Gently push skin towards the base of penis.

Personal Care Skills

Hold the penis by the shaft and wash in a circular motion from the tip down to the base. Use a clean area of washcloth or clean washcloth for each stroke. Rinse the penis. Then wash the scrotum and groin. The groin is the area from the pubis to the upper thighs. Rinse and pat dry. If resident is uncircumcised, gently return foreskin to normal position. Ask the resident to turn on his side. Wash, rinse, and dry buttocks and anal area. Cleanse the anal area without contaminating the perineal area.

14. Turn resident on his side away from you. Remove the wet protective pad after drying buttocks.

15. Place a dry protective pad underneath the resident.

    Keeps linen from getting wet.

16. Reposition resident.

17. Empty, rinse, and wipe basin and return to proper storage.

18. Place soiled clothing and linens in appropriate containers.

19. Dispose of soiled protective pads in proper containers.

20. Remove and dispose of gloves properly.

21. Return bed to appropriate level. Put signaling device within resident's reach.

    Lowering the bed provides for safety. Signaling device allows resident to communicate with staff as necessary.

22. Wash hands.

    Provides for infection control.

23. Report any changes in resident to the nurse.

    Provides nurse with information to assess resident.

24. Document procedure according to facility guidelines.

    What you write is a legal record of what you did. If you don't document it, legally it didn't happen.

👁 *When washing perineal area, use a clean area of the washcloth or clean washcloth for each stroke.*

Constipation is the inability to have a bowel movement. An enema or suppository may be ordered to assist. An **enema** is a specific amount of water flowed into the colon to eliminate stool. A **suppository** is a medication given rectally to cause a bowel movement. If allowed and trained to do so, follow your facility's policy on assisting with these treatments.

❤ *A low-fiber diet, decreased fluid intake, inactivity, medications, aging, and certain diseases are common causes of constipation.*

Unit 7: Identify guidelines for good skin care

Bony prominences are areas of the body where the bone lies close to the skin. The skin here is at a much higher risk for skin breakdown. These areas include elbows, shoulder blades, tailbone, hip bones, ankles, heels, and the back of the neck and head.

Other areas at risk are the ears, the area under the breasts, and the scrotum (Fig. 5-35). The pressure on these areas reduces circulation, decreasing the amount of oxygen the cells receive. Warmth and moisture also contribute to skin breakdown. Once the surface of the skin is weakened, pathogens can invade and cause infection. When infection occurs, the healing process slows down.

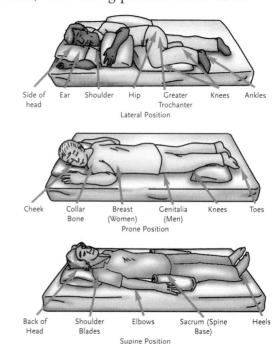

| Side of head | Ear | Shoulder | Hip | Greater Trochanter | Knees | Ankles |

Lateral Position

| Cheek | Collar Bone | Breast (Women) | Genitalia (Men) | Knees | Toes |

Prone Position

| Back of Head | Shoulder Blades | Elbows | Sacrum (Spine Base) | Heels |

Supine Position

Fig. 5-35. Pressure sore danger zones.

When skin begins to break down, it becomes pale, white, or a reddened color. Darker skin may appear purple. The resident may also complain of tingling or burning in the area. This discoloration does not go away, even when the resident's position is changed. If pressure is allowed to continue, the area will further deteriorate, or break down. The resulting wound is called a **pressure sore**, **bed sore**, or **decubitus ulcer**.

Once a pressure sore forms, it can get bigger, deeper, and infected. Approximately 90% of pressure sores in nursing homes develop within the first three weeks of admission. Pressure sores are painful and difficult to heal. They can lead to life-threatening infection. Prevention is very important (Fig. 5-36).

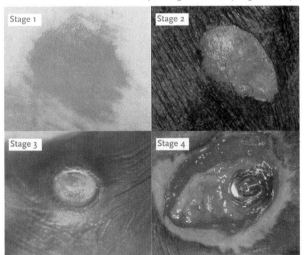

Fig. 5-36. Pressure sores are categorized by four stages.

OBSERVING AND REPORTING
Resident's Skin

- pale, white or reddened, or purple areas, or blistered or bruised areas on the skin
- complaints of tingling, warmth, or burning of the skin
- dry or flaking skin
- itching or scratching
- rash or any skin discoloration
- swelling
- blisters
- fluid or blood draining from skin
- broken skin
- wounds or ulcers on the skin
- changes in an existing wound or ulcer (size, depth, drainage, color, odor)
- redness or broken skin between toes or around toenails

GUIDELINES
Basic Skin Care

- Report changes you observe in a resident's skin.
- Provide regular care for skin to keep it clean and dry. When complete baths are not given or taken every day, check the resident's skin and provide skin care daily.
- Reposition immobile residents frequently (at least every two hours).
- Change clothing and linens as often as needed for incontinent residents. Check on them every two hours or as needed.
- Avoid scratching or irritating the skin in any way. Report to your supervisor if a resident wears shoes or slippers that cause blisters or sores.
- Massage the skin frequently, using light, circular strokes to increase circulation. Use little or no pressure on bony areas.
- Do not massage a white, red, or purple area or put any pressure on it. Massage the healthy skin and tissue surrounding the area.
- Be careful during transfers to avoid pulling or tearing fragile skin.

For residents who are not mobile or cannot change positions easily, remember the following points:

- Keep the bottom sheet tight and free from wrinkles and the bed free from crumbs.

Personal Care Skills

- Avoid pulling the resident across sheets during transfers or repositioning. This causes shearing, or pressure, when the surfaces rub against each other.

- Place a sheepskin, chamois skin, or bed pad under the back and buttocks to absorb moisture or perspiration that may accumulate and to protect the skin from irritating bed linens (Fig. 5-37).

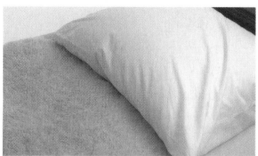

Fig. 5-37. A sheepskin or chamois skin may be placed to help absorb moisture. (Photo courtesy of Briggs Corporation)

- Relieve pressure under bony prominences. Place foam rubber or sheepskin pads under them. Heel and elbow protectors made of foam and sheepskin are available (Fig. 5-38).

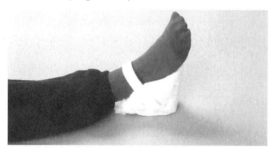

Fig. 5-38. Heel and elbow protectors made of sheepskin and foam are available. (Photo courtesy of Briggs Corporation)

- A bed or chair can be made softer with flotation pads or an egg crate mattress.

- Use a bed cradle to keep top sheets from rubbing the resident's skin. A bed cradle is made of metal.

- Residents seated in chairs or wheelchairs need to be repositioned frequently, too.

Many positioning devices are available to help make residents more comfortable and safe.

GUIDELINES
Using Positioning Devices

- Backrests can be regular pillows or special wedge-shaped foam pillows.

- Bed cradles are used to keep the bed covers from pushing down on resident's feet.

- Use **draw sheets**, or turning sheets, under residents who are unable to assist with turning in bed, lifting, or moving up in bed (Fig. 5-39). Draw sheets help prevent skin damage caused by shearing.

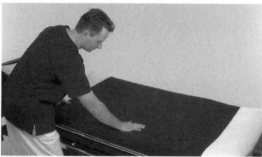

Fig. 5-39. A draw sheet.

- Footboards are padded boards placed against the resident's feet to keep them flexed.

- Hand rolls keep the fingers from curling tightly.

The survey team will look to see that staff have taken all necessary steps to prevent pressure sores. This includes turning and positioning residents, helping residents with eating and drinking, and managing episodes of incontinence.

A back rub can help relax your resident and make him more comfortable and increase circulation. Back rubs are often given after baths.

Giving a back rub

Equipment: cotton blanket or towel, lotion

1. **Wash hands.**
   Provides for infection control.

2. **Identify yourself to resident by name. Address resident by name.**

Resident has right to know identity of his or her caregiver. Addressing resident by name shows respect and establishes correct identification.

3. **Explain procedure to resident, speaking clearly, slowly, and directly, maintaining face-to-face contact whenever possible.**
   Promotes understanding and independence.

4. **Provide for resident's privacy during procedure with curtain, screen, or door.**
   Maintains resident's right to privacy and dignity.

5. **Adjust bed to a safe working level, usually waist high.**
   Prevents injury to you and to resident.

6. **Position resident lying on his stomach. If this is uncomfortable, have resident lie on his side. Cover with a cotton blanket. Expose back to the top of the buttocks. Back rubs can also be given with the resident sitting up (Fig. 5-40).**

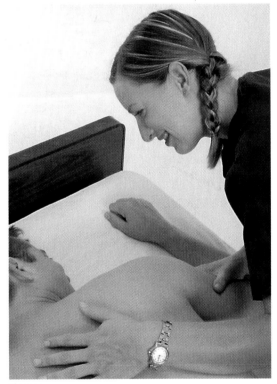

Fig. 5-40.

7. **Pour lotion on your hands. Rub them together. Always put lotion on your hands rather than directly on resident's skin. Warm lotion by putting lotion bottle in warm water for five minutes. Run your hands under warm water.**
   Increases resident's comfort.

8. **Place hands on each side of upper part of the buttocks. Make long, smooth upward strokes with both hands along each side of** the spine, up to the shoulders (Fig. 5-41). **Circle hands outward. Move back along outer edges of the back. At buttocks, make another circle and move hands back up to the shoulders. Without taking hands from resident's skin, repeat this motion for three to five minutes.**
   Long upward strokes release muscle tension. Circular strokes increase circulation in muscle areas.

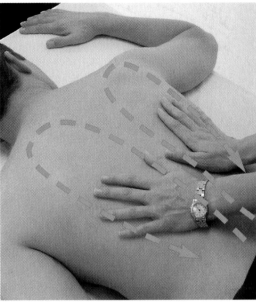

Fig. 5-41.

9. **Make kneading motions with the first two fingers and thumb of each hand. Place them at base of the spine. Move upward together along each side of the spine, applying gentle downward pressure with fingers and thumbs. Follow same direction as with the long smooth strokes, circling at shoulders and buttocks (Fig. 5-42).**

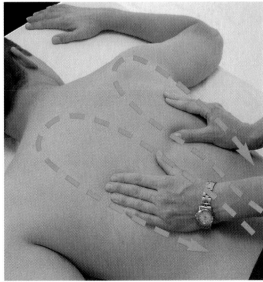

Fig. 5-42.

Personal Care Skills

10. **Gently massage bony areas (spine, shoulder blades, hip bones) with circular motions of fingertips. If any of these areas are red, massage around them rather than on them.**
    Redness indicates that skin is already irritated and fragile.

11. **Finish with some long, smooth strokes.**

12. **Dry the back if extra lotion remains on it.**

13. **Remove blanket and towel.**

14. **Assist the resident with getting dressed.**

15. **Store supplies. Place soiled clothing and linens in appropriate containers.**

16. **Return bed to appropriate level.**
    Provides for resident's safety.

17. **Before leaving resident, place signaling device within resident's reach.**
    Allows resident to communicate with staff as necessary.

18. **Wash hands.**
    Provides for infection control.

19. **Report any changes in resident to the nurse.**
    Provides nurse with information to assess resident.

20. **Document procedure according to facility guidelines.**
    What you write is a legal record of what you did. If you don't document it, legally it didn't happen.

Unit 8: **Explain the guidelines for safely transferring and positioning residents**

One of the most important considerations during resident transfers is safety. In 2002, the Occupational Safety and Health Administration (OSHA) announced new ergonomic guidelines for transferring residents. **Ergonomics** is the practice of designing equipment and work tasks to suit the worker's abilities. OSHA now recommends that manual lifting of residents should be minimized in all cases and eliminated when possible. Manual lifting, transferring, and repositioning of residents are tasks that have been associated with increased risks of pain and injury. For facilities, this means purchasing equipment to help aides perform these tasks. For aides, this means using provided equipment properly. When transferring and positioning, follow these safety guidelines:

Wheelchairs

- Learn how a wheelchair works. You should know how to apply and release the brake and how to operate the footrests. The wheelchair should be locked before assisting a resident into or out of it (Fig. 5-43). After a transfer, a wheelchair should be unlocked.

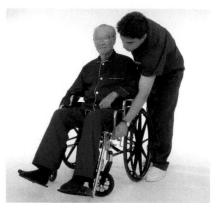

Fig. 5-43. You must always lock the wheelchair before a resident gets into or out of it.

- Make sure the resident is safe and comfortable during transfers.

- Ask the resident how you can assist with wheelchairs. Some residents may only want you to bring the chair to the bedside, while others may want you to be more involved.

Mechanical Lifts

You may assist the resident with many types of transfers using the mechanical or hydraulic lift if you are trained to do so. This equipment avoids wear and tear on your body. Lifts help prevent injury to you and the resident.

- Never use equipment you have not been trained to use. You or your resident could get hurt if you use lifting equipment improperly.

- There are many different types of mechanical lifts. You must be trained on the specific lift you will be using. Using these devices helps prevent common workplace injuries. Please understand and use provided equipment (Fig. 5-44).

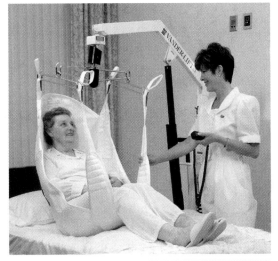

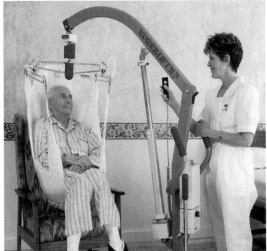

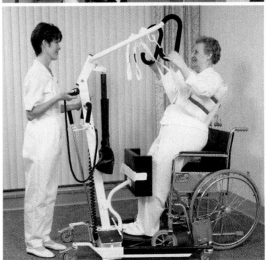

Fig. 5-44. Today, there are lifts for transferring both completely dependent residents and residents who can bear some weight. (Photo courtesy of VANCARE Inc., 800-694-4525)

Some transfers require use of additional devices. A **transfer belt**, or **gait belt**, is used to assist residents who are able to walk but are weak, unsteady, or uncoordinated. The belt is made of canvas or other heavy material. It sometimes has handles and fits around the resident's waist outside her clothing. When putting a belt on, leave enough room to insert two fingers into the belt (Fig. 5-45). The transfer belt is a safety device that gives you something firm to hold on to. Transfer belts may not be used if a resident has fragile bones or has had recent fractures.

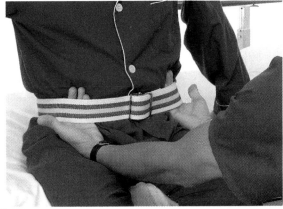

Fig. 5-45.

A sliding or transfer board may be used to help transfer residents who are unable to bear weight on their legs. Slide boards can be used for almost any transfer that involves moving from one sitting position to another. For example, slide boards can be helpful for transfers from a bed to a chair (Fig. 5-46).

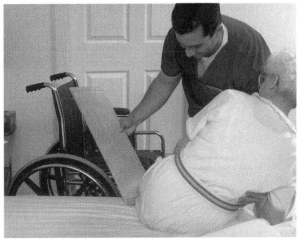

Fig. 5-46.

Falls

When a resident falls:

• Widen your stance and bring the resident's body close to you to break the fall. Bend your knees and support the resident as you lower her to the floor (Fig. 5-47).

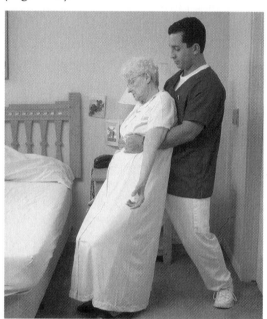

Fig. 5-47. Maintaining a wide base of support will help you assist a falling resident.

• Do not try to reverse or stop a fall. You or the resident can suffer worse injuries if you try to stop it rather than break it.

• Call for help. Do not attempt to get the resident up after the fall. Follow your facility's policies and procedures. Take resident's vital signs. Report the fall to nurse so that the incident report can be prepared.

Assisting resident to move up in bed

1. **Wash hands.**
   Provides for infection control.

2. **Identify yourself to resident by name. Address resident by name.**
   Resident has right to know identity of his or her caregiver. Addressing resident by name shows respect and establishes correct identification.

3. **Explain procedure to resident, speaking clearly, slowly, and directly, maintaining face-to-face contact whenever possible.**
   Promotes understanding and independence.

4. **Provide for resident's privacy during procedure with curtain, screen, or door.**
   Maintains resident's right to privacy and dignity.

5. **Adjust bed to a safe working level, usually waist high.**
   Prevents injury to you and to resident.

6. **Lower the head of bed. Move pillow to head of the bed. Lock bed wheels.**
   When bed is flat, resident can be moved without working against gravity. Pillow prevents injury should resident hit the head of bed.

7. **Lower the side rail (if not already lowered) on side nearest you.**

8. **Stand alongside bed with feet apart, facing the resident.**

9. **Place one arm under resident's shoulder blades and the other arm under resident's thighs.**
   Putting your arm under resident's neck could cause injury.

10. **Instruct resident to bend knees, brace feet on mattress, and push feet on the count of three.**
    Enables resident to help as much as possible and reduces strain on you.

11. **On signal, shift body weight to move resident, while resident pushes with her feet (Fig. 5-48).**
    Communicating helps resident help you.

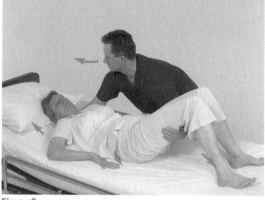

Fig. 5-48.

12. **Place pillow under resident's head.**
    Provides for resident's comfort.

13. **Return bed to appropriate level.**
    Lowering the bed provides for resident's safety.

14. **Before leaving resident, place signaling device within resident's reach.**
    Allows resident to communicate with staff as necessary.

15. **Wash hands.**
    Provides for infection control.

16. **Report any changes in resident to the nurse.**
    Provides nurse with information to assess resident.

17. **Document procedure according to facility guidelines.**
    What you write is a legal record of what you did. If you don't document it, legally it didn't happen.

Moving a resident to the side of the bed

1. **Wash hands.**
   Provides for infection control.

2. **Identify yourself to resident by name. Address resident by name.**
   Resident has right to know identity of his or her caregiver. Addressing resident by name shows respect and establishes correct identification.

3. **Explain procedure to resident, speaking clearly, slowly, and directly, maintaining face-to-face contact whenever possible.**
   Promotes understanding and independence.

4. **Provide for resident's privacy during procedure with curtain, screen, or door.**
   Maintains resident's right to privacy and dignity.

5. **Adjust bed to a safe working level, usually waist high.**
   Prevents injury to you and to resident.

6. **Lower the head of bed. Lock bed wheels (Fig. 5-49).**
   When bed is flat, resident can be moved without working against gravity.

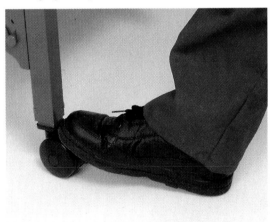

Fig. 5-49. Always lock the bed wheels before repositioning a resident in bed or transferring a resident to or from a bed.

7. **Gently slide your hands under the head and shoulders and move toward you (Fig. 5-50). Gently your slide hands under midsection and move toward self. Gently slide your hands under hips and legs and move toward self (Fig. 5-51).**
   Protects resident's skin.

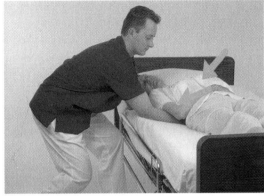

Fig. 5-50.

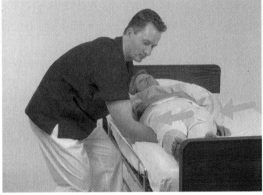

Fig. 5-51.

8. **Return bed to appropriate level.**
   Lowering the bed provides for resident's safety.

9. **Before leaving resident, place signaling device within resident's reach.**
   Allows resident to communicate with staff as necessary.

10. **Wash hands.**
    Provides for infection control.

11. **Report any changes in resident to the nurse.**
    Provides nurse with information to assess resident.

12. **Document procedure according to facility guidelines.**
    What you write is a legal record of what you did. If you don't document it, legally it didn't happen.

Turning a resident

1. **Wash hands.**
   Provides for infection control.

2. **Identify yourself to resident by name. Address resident by name.**
   Resident has right to know identity of his or her caregiver. Addressing resident by name shows respect and establishes correct identification.

3. **Explain procedure to resident, speaking clearly, slowly, and directly, maintaining face-to-face contact whenever possible.**
   Promotes understanding and independence.

Personal Care Skills

4. **Provide for resident's privacy during procedure with curtain, screen, or door.**
Maintains resident's right to privacy and dignity.

5. **Adjust bed to a safe working level, usually waist high.**
Prevents injury to you and to resident.

6. **Lower the head of bed. Lock bed wheels.**
When bed is flat, resident can be moved without working against gravity.

7. **Stand on side of bed opposite to where person will be turned. The far side rail should be raised.**

8. **Lower side rail nearest you if it is up.**

9. **Move resident to side of bed nearest you using previous procedure.**
Positions resident for turn.

10. **Cross resident's arm over his or her chest. Cross the leg nearest you over the far leg.**

11. *Moving resident away from you:*

    a. **Stand with feet approximately 12 inches apart. Bend your knees.**
    Reduces your risk of injury. Promotes good body mechanics.

    b. **Place one hand on the resident's shoulder and the other on the resident's hip nearest you.**

    c. **Gently push the resident toward the other side of the bed. Shift your weight from your back leg to your front leg (Fig. 5-52).**

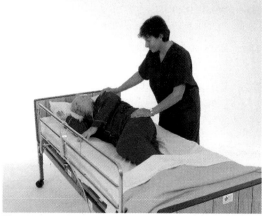

Fig. 5-52.

Moving resident toward you:

a. **Raise the side rail nearest you. Go to the other side and lower that side rail.**

b. **Stand with feet approximately 12 inches apart. Bend your knees.**
Reduces your risk of injury. Promotes good body mechanics.

c. **Place one hand on the resident's far shoulder and the other on the resident's far hip.**

d. **Gently roll the resident toward you (Fig. 5-53).**

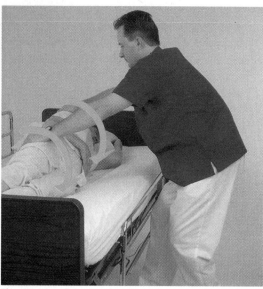

Fig. 5-53.

12. **Position resident properly. Proper body alignment requires:**

    head supported by pillow

    shoulder adjusted so resident is not lying on arm

    top arm supported by pillow

    back supported by supportive device

    top knee flexed

    top leg supported by supportive device with hip in proper alignment (Fig. 5-54)

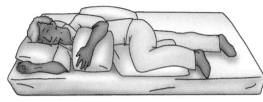

Fig. 5-54.

13. **Return bed to appropriate level.**
Lowering the bed provides for resident's safety.

14. **Before leaving resident, place signaling device within resident's reach.**
Allows resident to communicate with staff as necessary.

15. **Wash hands.**
Provides for infection control.

16. **Report any changes in resident to the nurse.**
Provides nurse with information to assess resident.

17. **Document procedure according to facility guidelines.**

    What you write is a legal record of what you did. If you don't document it, legally it didn't happen.

Logrolling a resident with one assistant

Logrolling means moving a resident as a unit, without disturbing the alignment of the body. The head, back and legs must be kept in a straight line. This is necessary in case of neck or back problems, spinal cord injuries, or back or hip surgeries. A draw sheet assists with moving. A draw sheet is an extra sheet placed on top of the bottom sheet when the bed is made.

Equipment: draw sheet

1. **Wash hands.**

   Provides for infection control.

2. **Identify yourself to resident by name. Address resident by name.**

   Resident has right to know identity of his or her caregiver. Addressing resident by name shows respect and establishes correct identification.

3. **Explain procedure to resident, speaking clearly, slowly, and directly, maintaining face-to-face contact whenever possible.**

   Promotes understanding and independence.

4. **Provide for resident's privacy during procedure with curtain, screen, or door.**

   Maintains resident's right to privacy and dignity.

5. **Adjust bed to a safe working level, usually waist high.**

   Prevents injury to you and to resident.

6. **Lower the head of bed. Lock bed wheels.**

   When bed is flat, resident can be moved without working against gravity.

7. **Lower the side rail closest to you.**

8. **Both co-workers stand on the same side of the bed. One person stands at the resident's head and shoulders. The other stands near the resident's midsection.**

9. **Place the resident's arms across his or her chest. Place a pillow between the knees.**

10. **Stand with feet approximately 12 inches apart. Bend your knees.**

    Reduces your risk of injury. Promotes good body mechanics.

11. **Grasp the draw sheet on the far side (Fig. 5-55).**

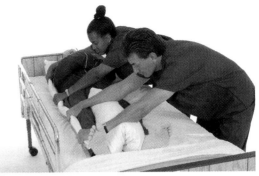

Fig. 5-55.

12. **On the count of three, gently roll the resident toward you. Turn the resident as a unit (Fig. 5-56).**

    Work together for your safety and the resident's.

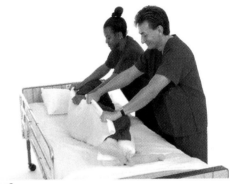

Fig. 5-56.

13. **Reposition resident comfortably.**

    Maintains alignment.

14. **Return bed to appropriate level.**

    Lowering the bed provides for resident's safety.

15. **Before leaving resident, place signaling device within resident's reach.**

    Allows resident to communicate with staff as necessary.

16. **Wash hands.**

    Provides for infection control.

17. **Report any changes in resident to the nurse.**

    Provides nurse with information to assess resident.

18. **Document procedure according to facility guidelines.**

    What you write is a legal record of what you did. If you don't document it, legally it didn't happen.

Assisting resident to sit up on side of bed

1. **Wash hands.**

   Provides for infection control.

2. **Identify yourself to resident by name. Address resident by name.**

   Resident has right to know identity of his or her

Personal Care Skills

caregiver. *Addressing resident by name shows respect and establishes correct identification.*

3. **Explain procedure to resident, speaking clearly, slowly, and directly, maintaining face-to-face contact whenever possible.**
   Promotes understanding and independence.

4. **Provide for resident's privacy during procedure with curtain, screen, or door.**
   Maintains resident's right to privacy and dignity.

5. **Adjust bed height to lowest position.**
   Allows resident's feet to touch floor when sitting. Reduces chance of injury if resident falls.

6. **Raise the head of bed to sitting position. Lock bed wheels.**
   Resident can move without working against gravity.

7. **Place one arm under resident's shoulder blades and the other arm under resident's thighs (Fig. 5-57).**
   Placing your arm under the resident's neck may cause injury.

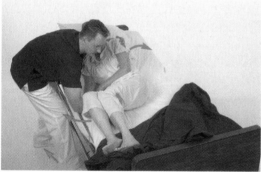

Fig. 5-57.

8. **On the count of three, slowly turn resident into sitting position with legs dangling over side of bed (Fig. 5-58).**
   Communicating helps resident help you.

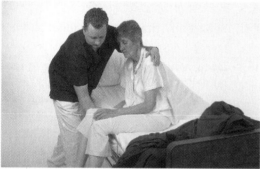

Fig. 5-58.

9. **Support for 10 to 15 seconds. Check for dizziness.**
   Change of position may cause dizziness due to a drop in blood pressure. If dizziness occurs, have resident lie down again. Report to the nurse.

10. **Assist resident to put on shoes or slippers.**
    Prevents sliding on floor and protects resident's feet from contamination.

11. **Move resident to edge of bed so feet are flat on floor.**
    Allows resident to be in stable position.

12. **Before leaving resident, place signaling device within resident's reach.**
    Allows resident to communicate with staff as necessary.

13. **Wash hands.**
    Provides for infection control.

14. **Report any changes in resident to the nurse.**
    Provides nurse with information to assess resident.

15. **Document procedure according to facility guidelines.**
    What you write is a legal record of what you did. If you don't document it, legally it didn't happen.

Transferring a resident from bed to wheelchair

Equipment: wheelchair, transfer belt, non-skid footwear

1. **Wash hands.**
   Provides for infection control.

2. **Identify yourself to resident by name. Address resident by name.**
   Resident has right to know identity of his or her caregiver. Addressing resident by name shows respect and establishes correct identification.

3. **Explain procedure to resident, speaking clearly, slowly, and directly, maintaining face-to-face contact whenever possible.**
   Promotes understanding and independence.

4. **Provide for resident's privacy during procedure with curtain, screen, or door.**
   Maintains resident's right to privacy and dignity.

5. **Position wheelchair close to bed with arm of the wheelchair almost touching the bed. Wheelchair should be placed on resident's stronger, or unaffected, side.**
   Unaffected side supports weight.

6. **Fold up wheelchair footrests. Lock both wheels on wheelchair and bed.**
   Wheel locks prevent chair and bed from moving.

7. **Adjust bed to its lowest level.**
   Prevents injury to you and to resident.

8. **Assist resident to sitting position with feet flat on the floor. (see procedure *Assisting resident to sit up on side of bed*.)**

9. **Put non-skid footwear on resident and securely fasten.**
Promotes resident's safety. Reduces risk of falls.

10. **With transfer (gait) belt:**

    a. Stand in front of resident.

    b. Stand with feet approximately 12 inches apart. Bend your knees.
    Reduces your risk of injury. Promotes good body mechanics.

    c. Place belt around resident's waist. Grasp belt on both sides.

    Without transfer belt:

    a. Stand in front of resident.

    b. Stand with feet approximately 12 inches apart. Bend your knees.
    Reduces your risk of injury. Promotes good body mechanics.

    c. Place your arms around resident's torso under the arms.

11. **Provide instructions to enable resident to assist in transfer. Instructions may include the following:**

    "When you start to stand, push with your hands against the bed."

    "Once standing, if you're able, you can take small steps in the direction of the chair."

    "Once standing, reach for the chair with one arm."

12. **With your legs, brace resident's lower extremities to prevent slipping (Fig. 5-59).**

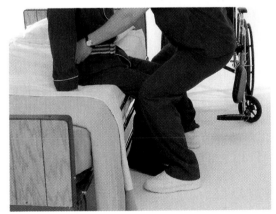

Fig. 5-59.

13. **Count to three to alert resident to begin transfer.**

14. **On signal, gradually assist resident to stand.**
Communicating helps resident help you.

15. **Assist resident to pivot to front of wheel-** chair with back of resident's legs against wheelchair.
Pivoting is safer than twisting.

16. **Lower resident into wheelchair.**

17. **Reposition resident with hips touching back of wheelchair and remove transfer belt, if used.**
Using full seat of chair is safest position.

18. **Position resident's feet on footrests.**
Protects feet and ankles.

19. **Before leaving resident, place signaling device within resident's reach.**
Allows resident to communicate with staff as necessary.

20. **Wash hands.**
Provides for infection control.

21. **Report any changes in resident to the nurse.**
Provides nurse with information to assess resident.

22. **Document procedure according to facility guidelines.**
What you write is a legal record of what you did. If you don't document it, legally it didn't happen.

👁 *You must lock the wheels on both the wheelchair and the bed before transferring.*

SIX

Basic Nursing Skills

Unit 1: Explain admission, transfer, and discharge of a resident

When a resident is admitted to a nursing home, the nursing assistant has an important role. This includes supporting residents emotionally. Moving into a nursing home is a big change. A resident may feel fear, loss, and uncertainty (Fig. 6-1). Because change is difficult, staff must communicate with new residents. Explain what to expect during the process. Answer any questions a resident has. Ask questions to find out a resident's personal preferences and routines.

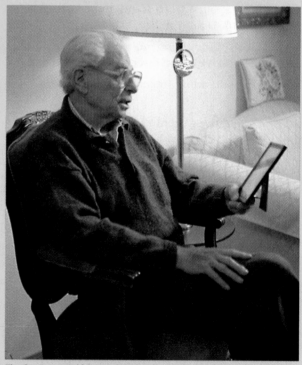

Fig. 6-1. A new resident may have just lost someone very close to him. Be supportive. Listen to him if he wants to talk.

Often, admission is the first time you meet a new resident. This is a time of first impressions. Make sure a resident has a good impression of you and your facility. Your facility will have a procedure for admitting residents to their new home. The following guidelines will make the experience as pleasant and successful as possible.

GUIDELINES
Admission

ⓖ Prepare the room before the resident arrives so he or she will feel expected and welcome. Know the condition of the resident. Know if he or she is bed-bound or is able to walk.

ⓖ Introduce yourself. Explain your position. Always address the person with his formal name until he tells you how he wants to be addressed.

ⓖ Never rush the process or the new resident. He should not feel as if he is an inconvenience.

ⓖ Make every effort to see that the new resident feels welcome and wanted.

ⓖ Explain day-to-day operations of the facility. Offer to take the resident on a tour if he has not had one (Fig. 6-2).

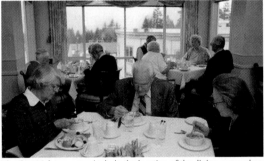

Fig. 6-2. Make sure you include the location of the dining room when taking a new resident on a tour.

ⓖ Introduce the resident to all staff members and residents you see (Fig. 6-3).

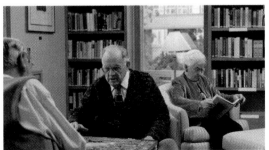

Fig. 6-3. Introduce new residents to all other residents you see.

ⓖ Handle personal possessions carefully and respectfully. These items are the special things he has chosen to bring with him. When setting up the room, ask about preferences. Place personal items where the resident wants them to be placed (Fig. 6-4).

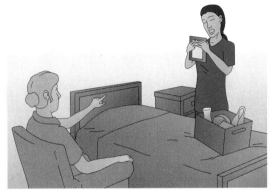

Fig. 6-4. Handle a resident's personal items carefully. Set up the room according to her preference.

ⓖ Follow the procedure of your facility regarding your tasks.

RⱯ Upon admission, residents must be informed of their rights and be provided with a written copy of these rights. This includes rights regarding personal funds and the right to file a complaint with the state survey agency.

Admitting a resident

Equipment: may include admission paperwork (checklist and inventory form), gloves and vital signs equipment

Often an admission kit will contain a urine specimen cup and transport bag, and personal care items, such as bath basin, water pitcher, drinking glass, toothpaste and soap.

1. **Wash hands.**
   Provides for infection control.

2. **Identify yourself to resident by name. Address resident by name.**
   Resident has right to know identity of his or her caregiver. Addressing resident by name shows respect and establishes correct identification.

3. **Explain procedure to resident, speaking clearly, slowly, and directly, maintaining face-to-face contact whenever possible.**
   Promotes understanding and independence.

4. **Provide for resident's privacy during procedure with curtain, screen, or door. If the family is present, ask them to step outside until the admission process is over.**

   Maintains resident's right to privacy and dignity.

5. **If part of facility procedure, perform the following (most of these are explained in more detail later in this chapter):**

   Take the resident's height and weight.

   Take the resident's vital signs.

   Obtain a urine specimen if required.

   Complete the paperwork, including an inventory of all the personal items.

   Assist the resident to put personal items away.

   Provide fresh water.

6. **Orient the resident to the room and bathroom. Explain how to work the bed (and television if there is one). Show the resident how to work the call light and explain its use.**

   Promotes resident's safety.

7. **Introduce the resident to his roommate, if there is one. Introduce other residents and staff.**

   Makes resident feel more comfortable.

8. **Before leaving the resident, place signaling device within resident's reach.**

   Allows resident to communicate with staff as necessary.

9. **Wash hands.**

   Provides for infection control.

10. **Document procedure according to facility guidelines.**

    What you write is a legal record of what you did. If you don't document it, legally it didn't happen.

Residents may be transferred to a different area within the facility, or, in cases of acute illness, may be transferred to a hospital. Change is difficult. This is especially true when a person has an illness or his or her condition gets worse. Make the transfer as smooth as possible for the resident. To lessen the stress, inform the resident of the transfer as soon as possible so he can begin to adjust to the idea. Explain how, where, when and why the transfer will occur.

For example, "Mrs. Jones, because you will be moving to a private room, you will be transferred to your new room in a wheelchair. This will happen on Wednesday morning around 10 a.m. The staff will take good care of you and your belongings. We will make sure you are comfortable. Do you have any questions?"

RA *Residents have the right to receive notice of any room or roommate change.*

Transferring a resident

Equipment: may include a wheelchair, cart for belongings, the medical record, all of the resident's personal care items

1. **Wash hands.**

   Provides for infection control.

2. **Identify yourself to resident by name. Address resident by name.**

   Resident has right to know identity of his or her caregiver. Addressing resident by name shows respect and establishes correct identification.

3. **Explain procedure to resident, speaking clearly, slowly, and directly, maintaining face-to-face contact whenever possible.**

   Promotes understanding and independence.

4. **Provide for resident's privacy during procedure with curtain, screen, or door.**

   Maintains resident's right to privacy and dignity.

5. **Collect the items to be transferred onto the cart and take them to the new location. If the resident is going into the hospital, the facility may want the belongings placed in a temporary storage area.**

6. **Assist the resident into the wheelchair (stretcher may be used for some residents).**

7. **Introduce new residents and staff.**

   Makes resident feel more comfortable.

8. **Assist the resident to put personal items away.**

9. **Make sure that the resident is comfortable. Before leaving, place signaling device within resident's reach.**

   Allows resident to communicate with staff as necessary.

10. **Wash hands.**

    Provides for infection control.

11. **Report any changes in resident to the nurse.**

Provides nurse with information to assess resident.

12. **Document procedure according to facility guidelines.**
    What you write is a legal record of what you did. If you don't document it, legally it didn't happen.

The day of discharge is usually a happy day for a resident who is going home. You will need to collect the resident's belongings and pack them. Know the condition of the resident and if he will be using a wheelchair or stretcher for discharge. Ask the resident which personal care items you need to include. Be positive and assure the resident he is ready for this important change. He may have doubts about not being cared for at the facility anymore. Remind him that his doctor believes he is ready.

The nurse may cover important information with the resident and family. Some of the following areas may be discussed:

- future doctor or physical therapy appointments (Fig. 6-5)

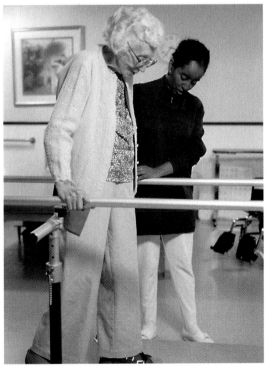

Fig. 6-5. After a resident is discharged, she may continue to receive physical therapy.

- medications
- the ambulation instructions from the doctor
- any restrictions on activities
- special exercises to keep the resident functioning at the highest level
- any special nutrition or dietary requirements
- community resources for assistance

Discharging a resident

Equipment: may include a wheelchair, cart for belongings, the discharge paperwork, including the inventory list done on admission, all of the resident's personal care items

1. **Wash hands.**
   Provides for infection control.

2. **Identify yourself to resident by name. Address resident by name.**
   Resident has right to know identity of his or her caregiver. Addressing resident by name shows respect and establishes correct identification.

3. **Explain procedure to resident, speaking clearly, slowly, and directly, maintaining face-to-face contact whenever possible.**
   Promotes understanding and independence.

4. **Provide for resident's privacy during procedure with curtain, screen, or door.**
   Maintains resident's right to privacy and dignity.

5. **Compare the checklist to the items there. If all items are there, ask the resident to sign.**

6. **Collect the items to be taken onto the cart and take them to pick-up area.**

7. **Assist the resident to dress and then into the wheelchair (stretcher may be used for some residents).**

8. **Assist the resident to say his goodbyes to the staff and residents.**

9. **Assist the resident into the wheelchair and transport him to the pickup area. Assist resident into vehicle. You are responsible for the resident until he or she is safely in the car.**

10. **Wash hands.**
    Provides for infection control.

Basic Nursing Skills

11. **Document procedure according to facility guidelines.**

What you write is a legal record of what you did. If you don't document it, legally it didn't happen.

📋 *The survey team will make sure that each resident has his or her rights protected and needs met during admission and/or discharge. This is true whether a resident is a private pay resident or on public aid. Staff must provide proper care and services regardless of who pays the bills.*

Unit 2: **Explain the importance of monitoring vital signs**

You will monitor, document, and report your residents' vital signs. Vital signs are important. They show how well the vital organs of the body, such as the heart and lungs, are working. You will develop excellent skills in measuring a resident's vital signs. They consist of the following:

- taking the body temperature
- counting the pulse
- counting the rate of respirations
- taking the blood pressure
- observing and reporting level of pain

Watching for changes in vital signs is important. It can indicate a resident's condition is worsening. Always notify the nurse if

- the resident is running a fever
- the resident has a respiratory or pulse rate that is too rapid or too slow
- the resident's blood pressure changes
- the resident's pain is worse or is not relieved by pain management

📋 *The survey team will make sure that staff take vital signs as indicated in the plan of care so that the resident's well-being and functioning are at their highest levels.*

Temperature

Body temperature is normally very close to 98.6° F (Fahrenheit) or 37° C (Celsius). Body temperature reflects a balance between the heat created by our bodies and the heat lost to the environment. Increases in body temperature may indicate an infection or disease. There are four sites for taking body temperature:

1. the mouth (oral)
2. the rectum (rectal)
3. the armpit (axillary)
4. the ear (tympanic)

The different sites require different thermometers. The site you use will depends on what kind of thermometer is available. There is a range of normal temperatures. Some people's temperatures normally run low. Others in completely good health will run slightly higher. Normal temperature readings also vary by the method used to take the temperature. A rectal temperature is generally considered to be the most accurate.

Normal Ranges for Adult Vital Signs		
Temperature:	Fahrenheit	Celsius
Oral	97.6°-99.6°	36.5°-37.5°
Rectal	98.6°-100.6°	37.0°-38.1°
Axillary	96.6°-98.6°	36.0°-37.0°
Pulse: 60-80 beats per minute		
Respirations: 12-20 respirations per minute		
Blood Pressure: Systolic 100-140, Diastolic 60-90		

Types of thermometers are

- Glass bulb (mercury) (Fig. 6-6)

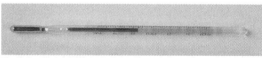

Fig. 6-6. A mercury glass thermometer.

- Battery-powered, digital (Fig. 6-7), or electronic (Fig. 6-8)

A 96. – 99
O 97. – 100
R 98. – 101

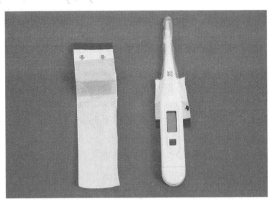

Fig. 6-7. A digital thermometer.

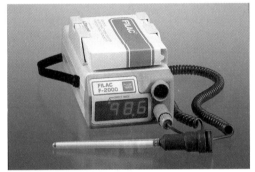

Fig. 6-8. An electronic thermometer.

- Tympanic (ear) (Fig. 6-9)

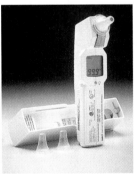

Fig. 6-9. A tympanic thermometer.

The point of a glass thermometer, known as the bulb end, contains mercury that will move along the length of the thin, hollow tube to register the temperature. Numbers on the thermometer let you read the temperature after it registers. Most thermometers show the temperature in degrees Fahrenheit (F), with each long line representing one degree and each short line representing two-tenths of a degree. Some thermometers show the temperature in degrees Celsius (C), with the long lines representing one degree and the short lines representing one-tenth of a degree. The small arrow points to the nor-

mal temperature: 98.6° F or 37° C.

When handling a mercury glass thermometer, handle it with care. Mercury is a hazardous substance. If the thermometer breaks, report it to the nurse immediately. When cleaning a mercury glass thermometer, wipe it with tissues first. Use cool water to clean it. Never use hot water. Hot water can heat the mercury and cause the thermometer to break. It may be cleaned or stored with a special disinfecting solution.

Taking and recording oral temperature

Equipment: glass, digital, or electronic thermometer, disposable plastic sheaths/covers for thermometers, tissues, pen and paper to record your findings

Do not take an oral temperature on a resident who has eaten or drunk fluids in the last 10–20 minutes.

1. **Wash hands.**
   Provides for infection control.

2. **Identify yourself to resident by name. Address resident by name.**
   Resident has right to know identity of his or her caregiver. Addressing resident by name shows respect and establishes correct identification.

3. **Explain procedure to resident, speaking clearly, slowly, and directly, maintaining face-to-face contact whenever possible.**
   Promotes understanding and independence.

4. **Provide for resident's privacy during procedure with curtain, screen, or door.**
   Maintains resident's right to privacy and dignity.

Using a glass thermometer:

5. **Hold thermometer by stem.**
   Holding the stem end prevents contamination of the bulb end. The thermometer reading must be below the resident's actual temperature.

6. **Before inserting oral thermometer in resident's mouth, shake oral thermometer down to below the lowest number. To shake the thermometer down, hold it at the side opposite the bulb with the thumb and two fingers. With a snapping motion of the wrist, shake the thermometer (Fig. 6-10).**

Stand away from furniture and walls while doing so.

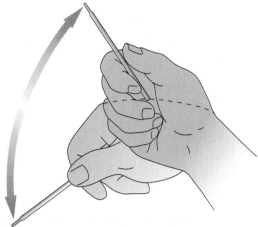

Fig. 6-10.

7. **Put on disposable sheath, if applicable. Insert bulb end of oral thermometer into resident's mouth, under tongue and to one side (Fig. 6-11).**
The thermometer measures heat from blood vessels under the tongue.

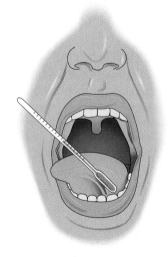

Fig. 6-11.

8. **Tell resident to hold oral thermometer in mouth with lips closed. Assist as necessary. Ask the resident not to bite down or to talk.**
The lips hold the thermometer in position. If broken, injury to the mouth and mercury poisoning may occur.

9. **Leave oral thermometer in place for ~~at least three minutes.~~** 5-8 minutes.
More time may be required if resident opens mouth to breathe or talk.

10. **Remove the thermometer. Wipe with tissue from stem to bulb or remove sheath. Dispose of tissue or sheath.**
Reduces contamination.

11. **Hold thermometer at eye level. Rotate until line appears. Read and record temperature.**
Record temperature immediately so you won't forget. Care plans are made based on your report.

12. **Clean oral thermometer and/or return it to container for used thermometers.**

Using a digital thermometer:

5. **Put on disposable sheath.**

6. **Turn on thermometer and wait until "ready" sign appears.**

7. **Insert end of digital thermometer into resident's mouth, under tongue and to one side.**

8. **Leave in place until thermometer blinks or beeps.**

9. **Remove the thermometer.**

10. **Read and record temperature on display screen.**
Record temperature immediately so you won't forget. Care plans are made based on your report.

11. **Using a tissue, remove and dispose of sheath.**
Reduces risk of contamination.

12. **Replace thermometer into case.**

Using an electronic thermometer:

5. **Remove probe from base unit.**

6. **Put on probe cover.**

7. **Insert end of electronic thermometer into resident's mouth, under tongue and to one side.**

8. **Leave in place until you hear a tone or see a flashing or steady light.**

9. **Read the temperature on the display screen.**

10. **Remove the probe. Press the eject button to discard the cover (Fig. 6-12).**

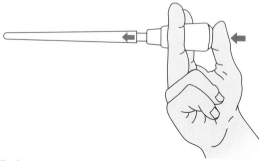

Fig. 6-12.

11. **Record temperature.**
Record temperature immediately so you won't forget. Care plans are made based on your report.

12. **Return the probe to the holder.**

Final steps:

13. **Before leaving resident, place signaling device within resident's reach.**
Allows resident to communicate with staff as necessary.

14. **Wash hands.**
Provides for infection control.

15. **Report any changes in resident to the nurse.**
Provides nurse with information to assess resident.

16. **Document procedure according to facility guidelines.**
What you write is a legal record of what you did. If you don't document it, legally it didn't happen.

Taking and recording axillary temperature

Equipment: glass thermometer, disposable plastic sheath, tissues, pen and paper to record your findings

1. **Wash hands.**
Provides for infection control.

2. **Identify yourself to resident by name. Address resident by name.**
Resident has right to know identity of his or her caregiver. Addressing resident by name shows respect and establishes correct identification.

3. **Explain procedure to resident, speaking clearly, slowly, and directly, maintaining face-to-face contact whenever possible.**
Promotes understanding and independence.

4. **Provide for resident's privacy during procedure with curtain, screen, or door.**
Maintains resident's right to privacy and dignity.

5. **Rinse thermometer in cool water and dry with clean tissue.**

6. **Remove resident's arm from sleeve of gown. Wipe axillary area with tissues.**
This removes moisture from axillary area.

7. **Hold thermometer at stem end and shake down to below the lowest number.**

8. **Put on disposable sheath, if applicable.**

9. **Place bulb end of thermometer in center of armpit and fold resident's arm over chest.**
Puts thermometer against blood vessels to get the reading.

10. **Hold in place for 10 minutes (Fig. 6-13).**

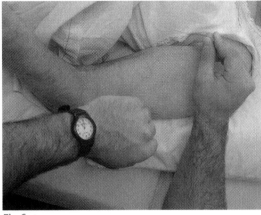

Fig. 6-13.

11. **Remove the thermometer. Wipe with tissue from stem to bulb or remove sheath (Fig. 6-14). Dispose of tissue or sheath.**
Reduces risk of contamination.

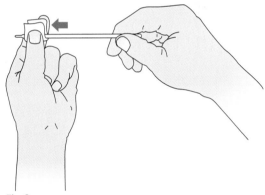

Fig. 6-14.

12. **Hold thermometer at eye level. Rotate until line appears. Read and record temperature.**
Record temperature immediately so you won't forget. Care plans are made based on your report.

13. **Clean thermometer and/or return it container for used thermometers.**

14. **Put resident's arm back into sleeve of gown.**

15. **Before leaving resident, place signaling device within resident's reach.**
Allows resident to communicate with staff as necessary.

16. **Wash hands.**
Provides for infection control.

17. **Report any changes in resident to the nurse.**
Provides nurse with information to assess resident.

18. **Document procedure according to facility guidelines.**
What you write is a legal record of what you did. If you don't document it, legally it didn't happen.

Basic Nursing Skills

Taking and recording rectal temperature

Equipment: rectal glass thermometer or digital thermometer, lubricant, gloves, tissue, disposable plastic sheath/cover, pen and paper to record your findings

1. **Wash hands.**
   Provides for infection control.

2. **Identify yourself to resident by name. Address resident by name.**
   Resident has right to know identity of his or her caregiver. Addressing resident by name shows respect and establishes correct identification.

3. **Explain procedure to resident, speaking clearly, slowly, and directly, maintaining face-to-face contact whenever possible.**
   Promotes understanding and independence.

4. **Provide for resident's privacy during procedure with curtain, screen, or door.**
   Maintains resident's right to privacy and dignity.

5. **Assist the resident to side-lying position (Fig. 6-15).**

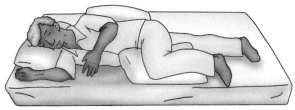

Fig. 6-15.

6. **Fold back linens to expose rectal area.**

7. **Put on gloves.**

8. *Glass thermometer*: **Hold thermometer by stem.**
   Digital thermometer: **Apply probe cover.**

9. *Glass thermometer*: **Shake thermometer down to below the lowest number.**

10. **Apply small amount of lubricant to bulb or probe cover (or apply pre-lubricated cover).**

11. **Gently insert thermometer into rectum one to one and a half inches.**

12. **Replace sheet over buttocks.**

13. *Glass thermometer*: **Hold thermometer in place for at least three minutes. Hold onto the thermometer at all times while taking a rectal temperature.**
    Digital thermometer: **Hold thermometer in place until thermometer blinks or beeps.**

Hold onto the thermometer at all times while taking a rectal temperature.

14. **Remove the thermometer. Wipe with tissue from stem to bulb or remove sheath. Dispose of tissue or sheath.**

15. **Read thermometer and record temperature.**
    Record temperature immediately so you won't forget. Care plans are made based on your report.

16. *Glass thermometer*: **Wash thermometer and/or return it to container for used thermometers.**
    Digital thermometer: **Throw away probe cover and return thermometer to storage area.**
    Reduces risk of contamination.

17. **Remove and dispose of gloves.**

18. **Assist resident to a position of safety and comfort.**

19. **Before leaving resident, place signaling device within resident's reach.**
    Allows resident to communicate with staff as necessary.

20. **Wash hands.**
    Provides for infection control.

21. **Report any changes in resident to the nurse.**
    Provides nurse with information to assess resident.

22. **Document procedure according to facility guidelines.**
    What you write is a legal record of what you did. If you don't document it, legally it didn't happen.

Taking and recording tympanic temperature

Equipment: tympanic thermometer, disposable probe sheath/cover, pen and paper to record your findings

1. **Wash hands.**
   Provides for infection control.

2. **Identify yourself to resident by name. Address resident by name.**
   Resident has right to know identity of his or her caregiver. Addressing resident by name shows respect and establishes correct identification.

3. **Explain procedure to resident, speaking clearly, slowly, and directly, maintaining face-to-face contact whenever possible.**
   Promotes understanding and independence.

4. **Provide for resident's privacy during procedure with curtain, screen, or door.**
   Maintains resident's right to privacy and dignity.

5.   **Put a disposable sheath over earpiece of the thermometer.**

Protects equipment. Reduces risk of contamination.

6.   **Insert the covered probe into the ear canal and press the button (Fig. 6-16).**

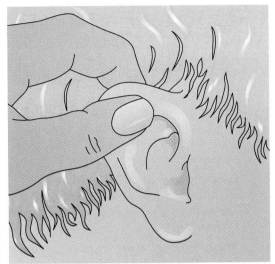

Fig. 6-16. Gently pull up/back on the outer edge of the ear before inserting the thermometer.

7.   **Hold thermometer in place until thermometer blinks or beeps.**

8.   **Read and record temperature.**

Record temperature immediately so you won't forget. Care plans are made based on your report.

9.   **Dispose of sheath. Return thermometer to storage area.**

10. **Before leaving resident, place signaling device within resident's reach.**

Allows resident to communicate with staff as necessary.

11. **Wash hands.**

Provides for infection control.

12. **Report any changes in resident to the nurse.**

Provides nurse with information to assess resident.

13. **Document procedure according to facility guidelines.**

What you write is a legal record of what you did. If you don't document it, legally it didn't happen.

Pulse

The pulse is essentially the number of heartbeats per minute. The beat that you feel at certain pulse points in the body represents the wave of blood moving as a result of the heart pumping. The most common site for checking the pulse is on the inside of the

wrist, where the radial artery runs just beneath the skin. This is called the **radial pulse**.

The brachial pulse is the pulse inside of the elbow, about 1–1½ inches above the elbow. The radial and brachial pulse are involved in taking blood pressure. Blood pressure is explained later in this chapter. Other common pulse sites are shown in Fig. 6-17.

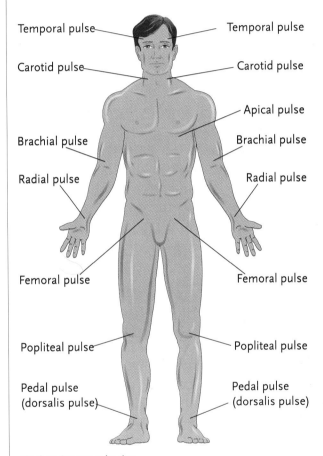

Fig. 6-17. Common pulse sites.

For adults, the normal pulse rate is 60–100 beats per minute. Small children have more rapid pulses, in the range of 100–120 beats per minute. A newborn baby's pulse may be as high as 120–160 beats per minute. Many things can affect the pulse rate, including exercise, fear, anger, anxiety, heat, medications, and pain. An unusually high or low rate does not necessarily indicate disease. However, sometimes the pulse rate can be a signal that serious illness exists. For example, a rapid

Basic Nursing Skills

pulse may result from fever, infection, or heart condition. A slow or weak pulse may indicate dehydration, infection, or shock.

Respirations

Respiration is the process of breathing air into the lungs, or **inspiration**, and exhaling air out of the lungs, or **expiration**. Each respiration consists of an inspiration and an expiration. The chest rises during inspiration and falls during expiration.

The normal respiration rate for adults ranges from 12 to 20 breaths per minute. Infants and children have a faster respiratory rate. Infants can breathe normally at a rate of 30–40 respirations per minute. People may breathe more quickly if they know they are being observed. Because of this, count respirations immediately after taking the pulse. Keep your fingers on the resident's wrist or the stethoscope over the heart. Do not make it obvious that you are observing the resident's breathing.

Taking and recording radial pulse, and counting and recording respirations

Equipment: watch with a second hand, pen and paper to record your findings

1. **Wash hands.**
    Provides for infection control.

2. **Identify yourself to resident by name. Address resident by name.**
    Resident has right to know identity of his or her caregiver. Addressing resident by name shows respect and establishes correct identification.

3. **Explain procedure to resident, speaking clearly, slowly, and directly, maintaining face-to-face contact whenever possible.**
    Promotes understanding and independence.

4. **Provide for resident's privacy during procedure with curtain, screen, or door.**
    Maintains resident's right to privacy and dignity.

5. **Place fingertips on thumb side of resident's wrist to locate pulse (Fig. 6-18).**

6. **Count beats for one full minute.**

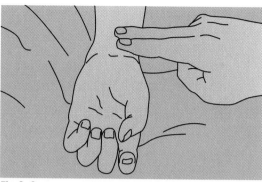
Fig. 6-18.

7. **Keeping your fingertips on the resident's wrist, count respirations for one full minute.**
    Count will be more accurate if resident does not know you are counting his respirations.

8. **Record pulse and respiration rate.**
    Record pulse and respiration rate immediately so you won't forget. Care plans are made based on your report.

9. **Before leaving resident, place signaling device within resident's reach.**
    Allows resident to communicate with staff as necessary.

10. **Wash hands.**
    Provides for infection control.

11. **Report any changes in resident to the nurse.**
    Provides nurse with information to assess resident.

12. **Document procedure according to facility guidelines.**
    What you write is a legal record of what you did. If you don't document it, legally it didn't happen.

Blood Pressure

Blood pressure is an important indicator of a person's health. Blood pressure is measured in millimeters of mercury (mm Hg). The measurement shows how well the heart is working. There are two parts of blood pressure, the systolic measurement and diastolic measurement.

In the **systolic** phase, the heart is at work, contracting and pushing blood out of the left ventricle. The reading you get shows the pressure on the walls of arteries as blood is pumped through the body. The normal range for systolic blood pressure is 100 to 140 mm Hg.

The second measurement reflects the **diastolic** phase—when the heart relaxes. The diastolic measurement is always lower than the systolic measurement. It shows the pressure in the arteries when the heart is at rest. The normal range for adults is 60 to 90 mm Hg.

When taking blood pressure, the first clear sound you will hear is the systolic pressure (top number). When the sound changes to a soft muffled thump or disappears, this is the diastolic pressure (bottom number). Blood pressure is recorded in a fraction. The systolic reading is on top and the diastolic reading is on the bottom (for example: 120/80).

Blood pressure is taken using a stethoscope and a blood pressure cuff, or sphygmomanometer (Fig. 6-19). Never measure blood pressure on an arm that has an IV, a dialysis shunt, or any medical equipment. Avoid a side that has a cast, recent trauma, or breast surgery (mastectomy).

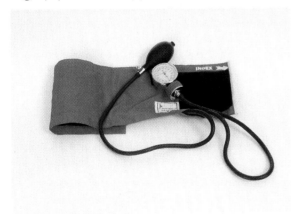

Fig. 6-19. A sphygmomanometer.

Taking and recording blood pressure (two-step method)

Equipment: sphygmomanometer (blood pressure cuff), stethoscope, alcohol wipes, pen and paper to record your findings

1. **Wash hands.**
   Provides for infection control.

2. **Identify yourself to resident by name.**

Address resident by name.
Resident has right to know identity of his or her caregiver. Addressing resident by name shows respect and establishes correct identification.

3. **Explain procedure to resident, speaking clearly, slowly, and directly, maintaining face-to-face contact whenever possible.**
   Promotes understanding and independence.

4. **Provide for resident's privacy during procedure with curtain, screen, or door.**
   Maintains resident's right to privacy and dignity.

5. **Position resident's arm with palm up. The arm should be level with the heart.**
   A false low reading is possible if arm is above heart level.

6. **With the valve open, squeeze the cuff to make sure it is completely deflated.**

7. **Place blood pressure cuff snugly on resident's upper arm, with the center of the cuff placed over the brachial artery (1-1½ inches above the elbow toward inside of elbow) (Fig. 6-20).**
   Cuff must be proper size and put on arm correctly so amount of pressure on artery is correct. If not, reading will be falsely high or low.

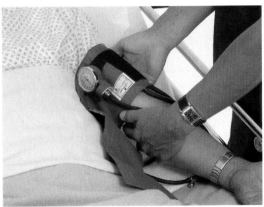

Fig. 6-20.

8. **Locate the radial (wrist) pulse with fingertips.**

9. **Close the valve (clockwise) until it stops. Inflate cuff, watching gauge.**

10. **Stop inflating when you can no longer feel the pulse. Note the reading. The number is an <u>estimate</u> of the systolic pressure.**
    This estimate helps you not to inflate the cuff too high later in this procedure. Inflating cuff too high is painful and may damage small blood vessels.

11. **Open the valve to deflate cuff completely.**
    An inflated cuff left on resident's arm can cause numbness and tingling.

12. **Write down the systolic reading.**

13. **Before using stethoscope, wipe diaphragm and earpieces of stethoscope with alcohol wipes.**
    Reduces pathogens, prevents ear infections and prevents spread of infection.

14. **Locate brachial pulse with fingertips.**

15. **Place earpieces of stethoscope in ears.**

16. **Place diaphragm of stethoscope over brachial artery.**

17. **Close the valve (clockwise) until it stops. Do not tighten it (Fig. 6-21).**
    Tight valves are too hard to release.

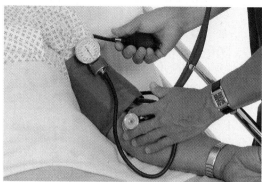

Fig. 6-21.

18. **Inflate cuff to 30 mm Hg above your estimated systolic pressure.**
    Inflating cuff too high is painful and may damage small blood vessels.

19. **Open the valve slightly with thumb and index finger. Deflate cuff slowly.**
    Releasing the valve slowly allows you to hear beats accurately.

20. **Watch gauge and listen for sound of pulse.**

21. **Remember the reading at which the first clear pulse sound is heard. This is the systolic pressure.**

22. **Continue listening for a change or muffling of pulse sound. The point of a change or the point the sound disappears is the diastolic pressure. Remember this reading.**

23. **Open the valve to deflate cuff completely. Remove cuff.**
    An inflated cuff left on resident's arm can cause numbness and tingling. If you must take blood pressure again, completely deflate cuff and wait 30 seconds. Never partially deflate a cuff and then pump it up again. Blood vessels will be damaged and reading will be falsely high or low.

24. **Record both systolic and diastolic pressures.**
    Record readings immediately so you won't forget. Care plans are made based on your report.

25. **Wipe diaphragm and earpieces of stethoscope with alcohol. Store equipment.**

26. **Before leaving resident, place signaling device within resident's reach.**
    Allows resident to communicate with staff as necessary.

27. **Wash hands.**
    Provides for infection control.

28. **Report any changes in resident to the nurse.**
    Provides nurse with information to assess resident.

29. **Document procedure according to facility guidelines.**
    What you write is a legal record of what you did. If you don't document it, legally it didn't happen.

Unit 3: Explain how to measure height and weight

You will check residents' weights and heights as part of your care. Height is checked less frequently than weight. Weight changes can be signs of illness. You must report **any** weight loss or gain, no matter how small.

Measuring and recording weight of an ambulatory resident

Equipment: standing scale, pen and paper to record your findings

1. **Wash hands.**
   Provides for infection control.

2. **Identify yourself to resident by name. Address resident by name.**
   Resident has right to know identity of his or her caregiver. Addressing resident by name shows respect and establishes correct identification.

3. **Explain procedure to resident, speaking clearly, slowly, and directly, maintaining face-to-face contact whenever possible.**
   Promotes understanding and independence.

4. **Provide for resident's privacy during procedure with curtain, screen, or door.**
   Maintains resident's right to privacy and dignity.

5. **Start with scale balanced at zero before weighing resident.**
   Scale must be balanced on zero for weight to be accurate.

6. **Assist resident to step onto the center of the scale.**

7. **Determine resident's weight. This is done by balancing the scale by making the balance bar level. Move the small and large weight indicators until the bar balances (Fig. 6-22).**

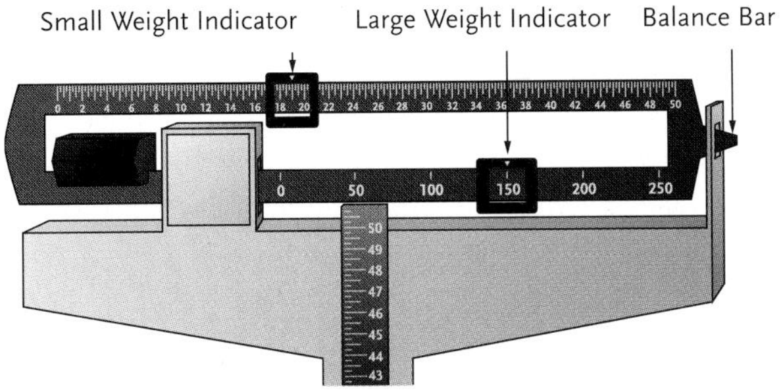

Small Weight Indicator   Large Weight Indicator   Balance Bar

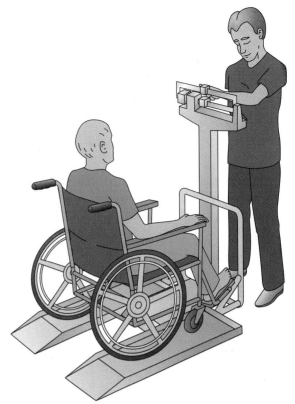

Fig. 6-22.

8. **Assist resident off scale before recording weight.**
   Protects against falls.

9. **Record weight.**
   Record weight immediately so you won't forget. Care plans are made based on your report.

10. **Before leaving resident, place signaling device within resident's reach.**
    Allows resident to communicate with staff as necessary.

11. **Wash hands.**
    Provides for infection control.

12. **Report any changes in resident to the nurse.**
    Provides nurse with information to assess resident.

13. **Document procedure according to facility guidelines.**
    What you write is a legal record of what you did. If you don't document it, legally it didn't happen.

Some residents will be unable to get out of a wheelchair easily. These residents may be weighed on a wheelchair scale. With this type of scale, wheelchairs are rolled onto the scale (Fig. 6-23). On some wheelchair scales, you will need to subtract the weight of the wheelchair before recording a resident's weight. In this case you must weigh the empty wheelchair and subtract the wheelchair's weight from the total. Some wheelchairs are marked with their weight.

Some residents will be unable to get out of bed. Weighing these residents requires a special scale (Fig. 6-24). Before using a bed

Fig. 6-23.

scale, know how to use it properly and safely. Follow your facility's procedure and any manufacturer's instructions.

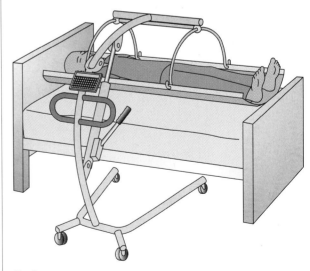

Fig. 6-24.

Measuring and recording height of an ambulatory resident

Equipment: standing scale, pen and paper to record your findings

1. **Wash hands.**
   Provides for infection control.

Basic Nursing Skills

2. **Identify yourself to resident by name. Address resident by name.**

   Resident has right to know identity of his or her caregiver. Addressing resident by name shows respect and establishes correct identification.

3. **Explain procedure to resident, speaking clearly, slowly, and directly, maintaining face-to-face contact whenever possible.**

   Promotes understanding and independence.

4. **Provide for resident's privacy during procedure with curtain, screen, or door.**

   Maintains resident's right to privacy and dignity.

5. **Assist resident to step onto scale.**

6. **Ask resident to stand straight. Assist as needed.**

   Ensures accurate reading.

7. **Pull up measuring rod from back side of scale. Gently lower measuring rod until it rests flat on resident's head (Fig. 6-25).**

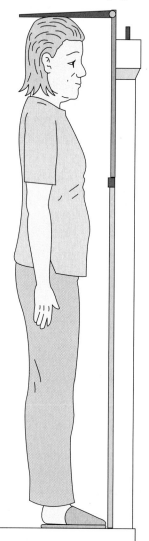

Fig. 6-25.

8. **Determine resident's height.**

9. **Assist resident off scale before recording height. Make sure measuring rod does not hit resident in the head while trying to help resident off the scale.**

   Protects resident from injury.

10. **Record height.**

    Record height immediately so you won't forget. Care plans are made based on your report.

11. **Before leaving resident, place signaling device within resident's reach.**

    Allows resident to communicate with staff as necessary.

12. **Wash hands.**

    Provides for infection control.

13. **Report any changes in resident to the nurse.**

    Provides nurse with information to assess resident.

14. **Document procedure according to facility guidelines.**

    What you write is a legal record of what you did. If you don't document it, legally it didn't happen.

The rod measures height in inches and fractions of inches. Record the total number of inches. If you have to convert a total number of inches into feet, remember that there are 12 inches in a foot.

If residents are unable to get out of bed, height can be measured by using a tape measure (Fig. 6-26). Position the resident lying straight in bed. Make marks on the sheet with a pencil at the top of the resident's head and at the bottom of the feet (Fig. 6-27). Measure the distance between the marks. Record the height.

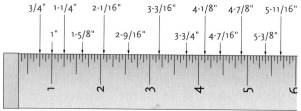

Fig. 6-26. A tape measure.

If the resident cannot lie in a straight position due to contractures, a tape measure can still be used to measure height. Start at the

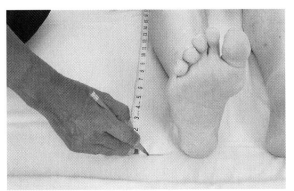

Fig. 6-27. Make marks on the sheet at the resident's head and feet.

top of the head and continue to the base of the heel, following the curves of the spine and legs. Total the number of inches and record them.

Unit 4: Explain restraints and how to promote a restraint-free environment

A **restraint** is a physical or chemical way to limit a person's movement. Examples of physical restraints are leg and arm ties, vests and jacket restraints, and chair or wheelchair bars. Side rails on a bed (Fig. 6-28) and special chairs that restrict movement (Fig. 6-29) are also considered physical restraints. Chemical restraints are medications given to control a person's behavior.

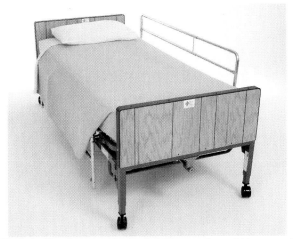

Fig. 6-28. Side rails are considered restraints because they restrict movement.

Generally, restraints are only used as a last resort. Restraints can never be used without a doctor's order. It is against the law for staff to apply restraints for staff convenience or to discipline a resident.

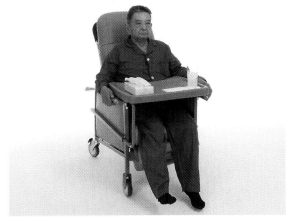

Fig. 6-29. When the tray table is attached, a geriatric chair is considered a restraint.

In nursing homes, restraints are sometimes ordered for the following reasons:

- To prevent a person from injuring self or other residents

- To prevent a person from pulling out tubing that is needed for treatment

There are many problems associated with restraints. Some of the negative effects of restraint use include the following:

- loss of dignity
- loss of independence
- reduced blood circulation
- stress on the heart
- incontinence
- weakened muscles and bones
- pressure sores
- increased agitation or depression
- poor self-esteem
- less activity, leading to poor appetite
- risk of suffocation
- pneumonia

Restraints have also caused death. Due to the serious problems caused by restraints, many facilities do not use them. Most have committed to make their facility restraint-free. This means they have developed ways to reduce the need for restraints. These methods are called **restraint alternatives**. A few of these alternatives include

- Assess medication use.

- Ambulate the resident when restless.

- Assist to the bathroom when restless.

- Assist in transferring to another bed or chair.

- Offer food or drink.

- Encourage exercise, activities, and independence (Fig. 6-30).

- Offer reading material: magazines, newspapers, etc.

- Assist back to bed for a nap.

- Offer a few minutes of one-on-one time with a caregiver.

- Decrease noise level.

- Give a repetitive task.

- Escort to social activities.

- Distract or redirect interest.

- Listen to soothing music.

- Answer call lights promptly.

- Provide familiar caregivers.

- Increase the number of caregivers using family and volunteers.

- Improve safety measures to prevent accidents and falls.

- Use a team approach to meeting resident's physical and psychological needs.

- Use postural devices to support and protect the residents' bodies.

- Offer training seminars to teach gentle approaches to difficult residents.

There are also several types of pads, belts, special chairs, and alarms that can be used instead of restraints. A few of these are shown below.

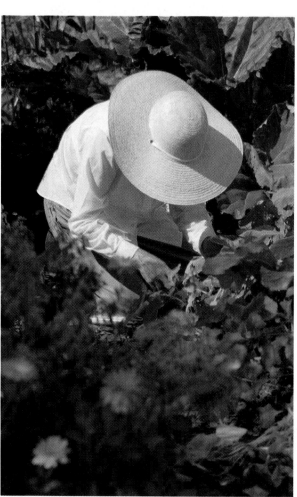

Fig. 6-30. Activities may help reduce the need for restraints.

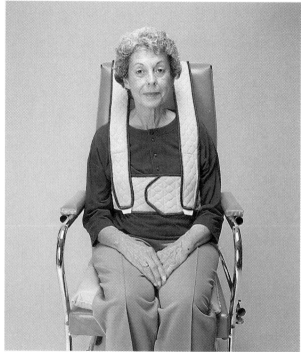

Fig. 6-31. A Posey Torso Support. (Photo courtesy of North Coast Medical, Inc., www.ncmedical.com, 800-821-9319)

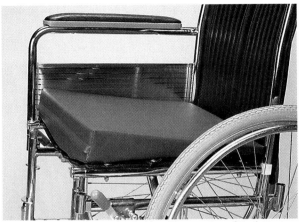

Fig. 6-32. A Posey Deluxe Wedge Cushion. (Photo courtesy of North Coast Medical, Inc., www.ncmedical.com, 800-821-9319)

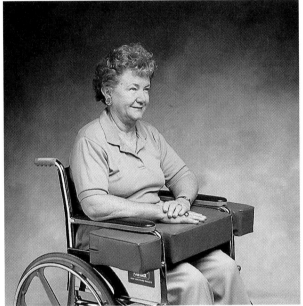

Fig. 6-33. A lap top cushion. (Photo courtesy of North Coast Medical, Inc., www.ncmedical.com, 800-821-9319)

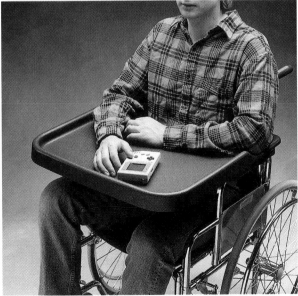

Fig. 6-34. A molded lap tray. (Photo courtesy of North Coast Medical, Inc., www.ncmedical.com, 800-821-9319)

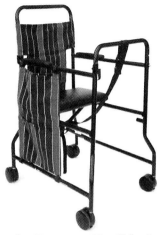

Fig. 6-35. A Merry Walker. (Photo courtesy Merry Walker Corporation, 815-678-3388)

[handwritten margin note: ⚑ = Calif. Title 22 reg's. will be in Red Cross test.]

When a resident is restrained, he or she has to be monitored continuously. The resident *[handwritten: to one hr. ⚑]* must be checked at least every 30 minutes. *[handwritten: and untied.]* Every two hours, ~~or as needed~~, the following must be done: *[⚑]*

- *[handwritten: Remove ⚑]* ~~Release~~ the restraint for at least ten minutes.

- Offer assistance with toileting. Check for episodes of incontinence. Provide incontinence care.

- Offer fluids.

- Check skin for irritation. Report any red areas to the nurse immediately.

- Reposition the resident.

- Ambulate resident if able.

If you are asked to apply a restraint, follow the manufacturer's instructions on how to do so.

The survey team will look for evidence that the facility is protecting a resident's right to be free from restraints. When a restraint is necessary, the team will look to see that staff protect the resident from harm.

Unit 5: Define fluid balance and explain intake and output (I&O)

Fluid balance is maintaining intake and output of fluids. It requires taking in the same

[sidebar: Basic Nursing Skills]

amount of fluid as the body puts out. Sometimes you will record what a resident consumes and voids. This is so the nurse or doctor can monitor the fluid balance. This information is recorded on an Intake/Output (I&O) sheet (Fig. 6-36). (See chapter 7 for more information on fluid balance.)

INTAKE AND OUTPUT RECORD

DATE	SHIFT	INTAKE (IN CC'S) ORAL	OUTPUT (IN CC'S) VOIDED	OUTPUT (IN CC'S) CATHETER	NUMBER OF INCONTINENT EPISODES (IF APPLICABLE)
	7-3				
	3-11				
	11-7				
	24 HR. TOTAL				
	7-3				
	3-11				
	11-7				
	24 HR. TOTAL				
	7-3				
	3-11				
	11-7				
	24 HR. TOTAL				
	7-3				
	3-11				
	11-7				
	24 HR. TOTAL				
	7-3				
	3-11				
	11-7				
	24 HR. TOTAL				
	7-3				
	3-11				
	11-7				
	24 HR. TOTAL				
	7-3				
	3-11				
	11-7				
	24 HR. TOTAL				

NAME-Last	First	Middle	Attending Physician	Record No.	Room/Bed

INTAKE AND OUTPUT RECORD

Fig. 6-36. A sample intake and output form.

Conversions

A cubic centimeter is a unit of measure and is equal to 1 milliliter.

1 oz. = 30 cc or 30 ml.

1 cup = 8 oz. = 240 cc

½ cup = 4 oz. = 120 cc

¼ cup = 2 oz. = 60 cc

Measuring and recording urinary output

Equipment: intake and output record, graduate (measuring container), gloves, pen and paper to record your findings

1. **Wash hands.**
   Provides for infection control.

2. **Put on gloves before handling bedpan/urinal.**

3. **Pour the contents of the bedpan or urinal into measuring container without spilling or splashing any of the urine.**

4. **Measure the amount of urine while keeping container level (Fig. 6-37).**
   Helps get accurate reading.

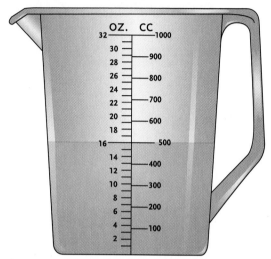

Fig. 6-37. A graduate is a measuring container.

5. **After measuring urine, empty contents of measuring container into toilet without splashing.**
   Reduces risk of contamination.

6. **Rinse measuring container and pour rinse water into toilet.**

7. **Rinse bedpan/urinal and pour rinse water into toilet.**

8. **Return bedpan/urinal and measuring container to proper storage.**

9. **Remove and dispose of gloves.**

10. **Wash hands before recording output.**
    Provides for infection control.

11. **Record contents of container in output column on sheet.**
    Record amount immediately so you won't forget. Care plans are made based on your report. What you write is a legal record of what you did. If you don't document it, legally it didn't happen.

12. **Report any changes in resident to the nurse.**
    Provides nurse with information to assess resident.

Catheter Care

A **catheter** is a tube used to drain urine from the bladder. A straight catheter does not remain inside the person. It is removed immediately after the urine is drained. An indwelling catheter remains inside the bladder for a period of time. The urine drains into a bag. Unit 6 has information on other kinds of tubing.

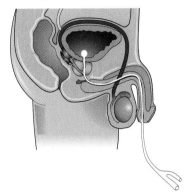

Fig. 6-38. An indwelling catheter (male).

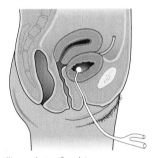

Fig. 6-39. An indwelling catheter (female).

GUIDELINES
Working with Residents Who Have Catheters

- The drainage bag must *always* be kept lower than the hips or bladder. Urine must never flow from the bag or tubing back into the bladder. That can cause infection.

- Tubing should be kept as straight as possible and should not be kinked.

- The genital area must be kept clean to prevent infection.

OBSERVING AND REPORTING
Catheter Care

- blood in the urine or any other unusual appearance

- catheter bag does not fill after several hours

- catheter bag fills suddenly

- catheter is not in place

- urine leaks from the catheter

- resident reports pain

- odor

Providing catheter care

Equipment: bath blanket, protective pad, bath basin, soap, bath thermometer, 2-4 washcloths, 1 towel, gloves

1. **Wash hands.**
   Provides for infection control.

2. **Identify yourself to resident by name. Address resident by name.**
   Resident has right to know identity of his or her caregiver. Addressing resident by name shows respect and establishes correct identification.

3. **Explain procedure to resident, speaking clearly, slowly, and directly, maintaining face-to-face contact whenever possible.**
   Promotes understanding and independence.

4. **Provide for resident's privacy during procedure with curtain, screen, or door.**
   Maintains resident's right to privacy and dignity.

5. **Adjust bed to a safe working level, usually waist high.**
   Prevents injury to you and to resident.

6. **Lower head of bed. Position resident lying flat on her back. Raise the side rail farthest from you.**

7. **Remove or fold back top bedding, keeping resident covered with bath blanket.**
   Promotes resident's privacy.

8. **Test water temperature with thermometer or your wrist and ensure it is safe. Water temperature should be 105° to 109° F. Have resident check water temperature. Adjust if necessary.**
   Resident's sense of touch may be different than yours; therefore, resident is best able to identify a comfortable water temperature.

9. **Put on gloves.**
   Prevents you from coming into contact with body fluids.

10. **Place clean protective pad under her buttocks. Ask the resident to flex her knees and raise the buttocks off the bed by pushing against the mattress with her feet.**
    Keeps linen from getting wet.

Basic Nursing Skills

11. **Expose only the area necessary to clean the catheter.**
    Promotes resident's privacy.

12. **Place towel or pad under catheter tubing before washing.**
    Helps keep linen from getting wet.

13. **Apply soap to wet washcloth.**

14. **Hold catheter near meatus to avoid tugging the catheter.**

15. **Clean at least four inches of catheter nearest meatus. Move in only one direction, away from meatus. Use a clean area of the cloth for each stroke.**
    Prevents infection.

16. **Rinse at least four inches of catheter nearest meatus. Move in only one direction, away from meatus (Fig. 6-40). Use a clean area of the cloth for each stroke.**

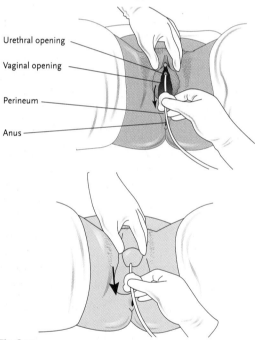

Urethral opening
Vaginal opening
Perineum
Anus

Fig. 6-40.

17. **Dispose of linen in proper containers.**

18. **Empty, rinse, and wipe basin and return to proper storage.**

19. **Remove and dispose of gloves.**

20. **Return bed to appropriate level. Put signaling device within resident's reach.**
    Lowering the bed provides for safety. Signaling device allows resident to communicate with staff as necessary.

21. **Place soiled clothing and linens in appropriate containers.**

22. **Wash hands.**
    Provides for infection control.

23. **Report any changes in resident to the nurse.**
    Provides nurse with information to assess resident.

24. **Document procedure according to facility guidelines.**
    What you write is a legal record of what you did. If you don't document it, legally it didn't happen.

👁 *When cleaning the catheter, move in one direction only, away from the genital area. Use a clean area of the cloth for each stroke.*

Collecting Specimens

You may be asked to collect a specimen from a resident. A **specimen** is a sample. Different types of specimens are used for different tests. You may be asked to collect these different types of specimens:

- Urine (clean catch/mid-stream or 24-hour)

- Stool (feces)

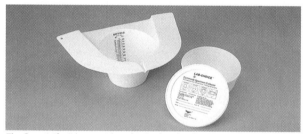

Fig. 6-41. A "hat" is a container that is placed under the toilet seat to collect specimens for residents who use the toilet.

Sputum specimens are collected to check for respiratory problems. **Sputum** is mucus coughed up from the lungs. Early morning is the best time to collect sputum.

Collecting a clean catch (mid-stream) urine specimen

Equipment: specimen kit with container, label, cleansing solution, gauze or towelettes, gloves, bedpan or urinal if resident cannot use the bathroom, plastic bag, washcloth, paper towel, towel, supplies for perineal care

Some residents will be able to collect their own specimens. Others will need your help. Be sure to explain exactly how the specimen must be collected. The specimen is called **mid-stream** because the first and last urine are not included in the sample.

1. **Wash hands.**
   Provides for infection control.

2. **Identify yourself to resident by name. Address resident by name.**
   Resident has right to know identity of his or her caregiver. Addressing resident by name shows respect and establishes correct identification.

3. **Explain procedure to resident, speaking clearly, slowly, and directly, maintaining face-to-face contact whenever possible.**
   Promotes understanding and independence.

4. **Provide for resident's privacy during procedure with curtain, screen, or door.**
   Maintains resident's right to privacy and dignity.

5. **Put on gloves.**
   Prevents you from coming into contact with body fluids.

6. **Open the specimen kit. Do not touch the inside of the container or the inside of the lid.**
   Prevents contamination.

7. **Using the towelettes or gauze and cleansing solution, clean the area around the urethra. For females, separate the labia and wipe from front to back along one side. Discard towelette/gauze. With a new towelette or gauze, wipe from front to back along the other labia. Using a new towelette or gauze, wipe down the middle.**

   For males, clean the head of the penis using circular motions with the towelettes or gauze. Clean thoroughly, changing towelettes/gauze after each circular motion and discarding after use. If the man is uncircumcised, pull back the foreskin of the penis before cleaning and hold it back during urination. Make sure it is pulled back down after collecting the specimen.
   Improper cleaning can infect urinary tract and contaminate the sample.

8. **Ask the resident to urinate into the bedpan, urinal, or toilet, and to stop before urination is complete.**

9. **Place the container under the urine stream and have the resident start urinating again. Fill the container at least half full. Have the resident finish urinating in bedpan, urinal, or toilet.**

10. **Cover the urine container with its lid. Wipe off the outside with a paper towel.**

11. **Place the container in a plastic bag.**
    Provides for safe transport.

12. **If using a bedpan or urinal, discard extra urine. Rinse and clean equipment, and store.**

13. **Remove and dispose of gloves. Wash hands. Help resident wash his or her hands at the sink or using the washcloth and towel.**
    Promotes infection control.

14. **Complete the label for the container with the resident's name, address, the date, and time.**

15. **Before leaving resident, place signaling device within resident's reach.**
    Allows resident to communicate with staff as necessary.

16. **Wash hands.**
    Provides for infection control.

17. **Report any changes in resident to the nurse.**
    Provides nurse with information to assess resident.

18. **Document procedure according to facility guidelines. Note amount and characteristics of urine.**
    What you write is a legal record of what you did. If you don't document it, legally it didn't happen.

Collecting a stool specimen

Equipment: specimen container and lid, 2 tongue blades, 2 pair gloves, bedpan and cover if resident cannot use the bathroom or commode, specimen pan if resident uses toilet or commode, 2 plastic bags, toilet tissue, laboratory slip, washcloth or towel, supplies for perineal care

Ask the resident to let you know when he or she can have a bowel movement. Be ready to collect the specimen.

1. **Wash hands.**
   Provides for infection control.

2. **Identify yourself to resident by name. Address resident by name.**
   Resident has right to know identity of his or her caregiver. Addressing resident by name shows respect and establishes correct identification.

3. **Explain procedure to resident, speaking clearly, slowly, and directly, maintaining face-to-face contact whenever possible.**
   Promotes understanding and independence.

4. **Provide for resident's privacy during procedure with curtain, screen, or door.**
   Maintains resident's right to privacy and dignity.

5. **Put on gloves.**
   Prevents you from coming into contact with body fluids.

Basic Nursing Skills

6. When the resident is ready to move bowels, ask him not to urinate at the same time and not to put toilet paper in with the sample. Provide a plastic bag to discard toilet paper separately.

Urine and paper ruin the sample.

7. Fit specimen pan to toilet or commode, or provide resident with bedpan. Leave the room and ask the resident to signal when he is finished with the bowel movement. Make sure call light is within resident's reach.

Promotes resident's privacy and dignity.

8. After the bowel movement, assist as necessary with perineal care. Help resident wash his or her hands at the sink or using the washcloth and towel. Make the resident comfortable. Remove gloves.

9. Wash hands again.

10. Put on clean gloves.

11. Using the two tongue blades, take about two tablespoons of stool and put it in the container. Cover it tightly.

12. Wrap the tongue blades in toilet paper and throw them away. Empty the bedpan or container into the toilet. Clean and store the equipment.

13. Complete the label for the container with the resident's name, address, the date, and time. Bag the specimen.

14. Remove and dispose of gloves.

15. Before leaving resident, place signaling device within resident's reach.

Allows resident to communicate with staff as necessary.

16. Wash hands.

Provides for infection control.

17. Report any changes in resident to the nurse.

Provides nurse with information to assess resident.

18. Document procedure according to facility guidelines. Note amount and characteristics of stool.

What you write is a legal record of what you did. If you don't document it, legally it didn't happen.

Unit 6: Explain care guidelines for different types of tubing

Residents are sometimes fed through a tube. This tube can travel through the nose and esophagus into the stomach. This is called a nasogastric tube. Or it can be placed through the skin directly into the stomach. This is called a gastrostomy (Fig. 6-42). Tube feedings are used when residents cannot swallow but can digest food. Conditions that may prevent residents from swallowing include coma, cancer, stroke, refusal to eat, extreme weakness, or a need for increased calories.

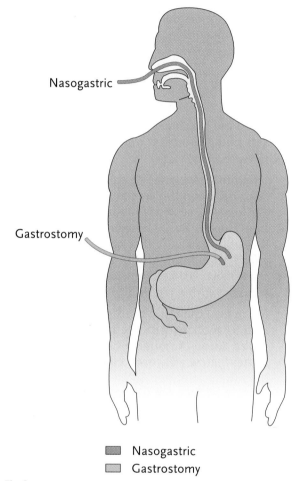

Nasogastric

Gastrostomy

■ Nasogastric
■ Gastrostomy

Fig. 6-42.

GUIDELINES
Working with Residents Who Have Gastric Tubes

• Tubing cannot be kinked. This means it cannot be curled, twisted, or bent. Check often for kinking. This is especially true when the resident turns in bed or walks.

• Make sure you know where tubing is when turning a resident. Check to make sure that a resident is not on top of the tubing.

- The tube is only inserted and removed by a doctor or nurse. If it comes out, report it immediately.

- A doctor will prescribe the type and amount of feeding. Do not place anything else into the tube. The feedings will be in a liquid form. The dietary department prepares them or they are prepackaged.

- Nursing assistants are not permitted to do the feedings. If the pump that delivers the feeding is not working or the alarm goes off, report it immediately.

- During the feeding, the resident should remain in a sitting position with the head of the bed elevated about 45 degrees.

- If your resident must remain in bed for long periods during feedings, provide good skin care to prevent pressure sores on the hips and sacral area.

- Provide frequent mouth care.

- If the tubing is inserted through the abdomen, watch the site for signs of infection. These include redness or drainage around the opening.

- If the tubing is inserted into the nose, secure the tubing to the nose and to the resident's gown. Securing the tape helps prevent irritation and pressure on the nose. Provide care to the nasal area for soreness and dryness.

Some residents with breathing difficulties may receive oxygen. It is more concentrated than what we breathe in the air. Oxygen is prescribed by a doctor. You should never stop, adjust, or administer oxygen for a resident. Oxygen may be piped into a resident's room through a central system. It may be in tanks or produced by an oxygen concentra-

tor. An oxygen concentrator changes air in the room into air with more oxygen.

Oxygen is a highly **combustible** gas. That means it can very easily explode or catch fire. Working around oxygen requires special safety precautions.

♥ *Oxygen is necessary for survival. Every cell needs oxygen. If a person stops breathing, death occurs within minutes. The respiratory system brings oxygen into the lungs and eliminates carbon dioxide.*

GUIDELINES
Working Safely Around Oxygen Equipment

- Remove all fire hazards from the room or area. Fire hazards include electric shavers, hair dryers, or other electrical appliances (Fig. 6-43).

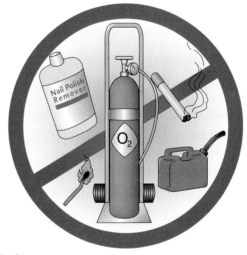

Fig. 6-43.

- Notify the nurse if a fire hazard is present and the resident does not want it removed.

- Post "No Smoking" and "Oxygen in Use" signs. Never allow smoking in the room or area where oxygen is used or stored.

- Never allow candles or other open flames around oxygen.

- Learn how to turn oxygen off in case of fire. Never adjust oxygen level.

🔢 Report if the nasal cannula or face mask is causing skin irritation. Check behind the ears for irritation from nasal cannula (Fig. 6-44).

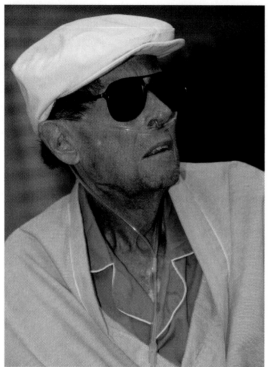

Fig. 6-44. A resident with a nasal cannula.

IV stands for **intravenous**, or into a vein. A resident with an IV is receiving medication, nutrition, or fluids through a vein. When a doctor prescribes an IV, a nurse inserts a needle into a vein. This allows direct access to the bloodstream. Medication, nutrition, or fluids either drip from a bag suspended on a pole or are pumped by a portable pump through a tube and into the vein (Fig. 6-45). Some residents with chronic conditions have

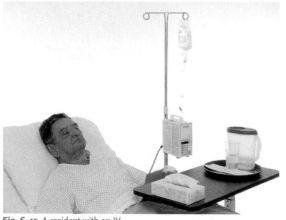

Fig. 6-45. A resident with an IV.

a permanent opening for IVs. This opening has been surgically created to allow easy access for IV fluids.

Nursing assistants never insert or remove IV lines. You will not be responsible for care of the IV site. Your only responsibility for IV care is to report and document any observations of changes or problems with the IV.

OBSERVING AND REPORTING
IVs

- The needle falls out or is removed.
- The dressing around the IV site is loose or not intact.
- Blood is in the tubing or around the site of the IV.
- The site is swollen or discolored.
- The resident complains of pain.
- The bag is broken, or the level of fluid does not seem to decrease.
- The IV fluid is not dripping.
- The IV fluid is nearly gone.
- The pump beeps, indicating a problem.

See chapter 5 for applying a gown on a resident with an IV.

Unit 7: **Explain the importance of sleep and perform proper bedmaking**

Sleep and rest are important needs that must be met. Sleep provides us with new cells and energy. Many elderly persons, especially those who are living away from their homes, have sleep and rest problems. Many things can affect sleep. Fear, anxiety, noise, diet, medications, and illness all affect sleeping patterns. Sharing a room with an unfamiliar person can disturb sleeping. When a resident complains of lack of sleep, staff should observe for things, such as:

- sleeping too much during the day

- too much caffeine late in the afternoon or evening

- dressing in night clothes during day instead of daytime wear

- eating too late at night

- refusing medication ordered for sleep

- taking new medications

- roommates who keep the TV or light on late at night

- pain

Bedmaking

Some residents spend much or all of their time in bed, so careful bedmaking is essential to comfort, cleanliness, and health. Linens should always be changed after personal care procedures such as bed baths. Also change them any time bedding or sheets are damp, soiled, or in need of straightening. It is important that residents' bed linens be changed frequently for three reasons:

1. Sheets that are damp, wrinkled, or bunched up under a resident are uncomfortable. They may prevent the resident from resting or sleeping well.

2. Microorganisms thrive in moist, warm environments. Bedding that is damp or unclean may encourage infection and disease.

3. Residents who spend long hours in bed are at risk for pressure sores. Sheets that do not lie flat under the resident's body increase this risk because they cut off circulation.

GUIDELINES
Bedmaking

- When collecting linen to make a bed, carry it away from your uniform. If linen touches your uniform, it becomes contaminated (Fig. 6-46).

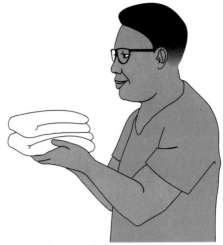
Fig. 6-46. Carry linen away from your uniform.

- Do not shake linen. It may spread airborne contaminants.

- Check linens for personal belongings, such as dentures, hearing aids, and glasses, before removing them.

If a resident cannot get out of bed, you must change the linens with the resident in bed. When making the bed, be careful to use a wide stance with knees bent. Avoid bending from the waist, especially when tucking sheets or blankets under the mattress. Mattresses can be heavy. Bend your knees to avoid injury. It is easier to make an unoccupied bed than one with a resident in it. If the resident can be moved to a chair or other comfortable spot, your job will be easier.

Making an occupied bed

Equipment: clean linen: mattress pad, fitted or flat bottom sheet, waterproof bed protector if needed, cotton draw sheet, flat top sheet, blanket(s), pillowcase(s), gloves (if you're going to be touching linens soiled with body fluids)

1. **Wash hands.**
   Provides for infection control.

2. **Identify yourself to resident by name. Address resident by name.**
   Resident has right to know identity of his or her caregiver. Addressing resident by name shows respect and establishes correct identification.

Basic Nursing Skills

3. **Explain procedure to resident, speaking clearly, slowly, and directly, maintaining face-to-face contact whenever possible.**
   Promotes understanding and independence.

4. **Provide for resident's privacy during procedure with curtain, screen, or door.**
   Maintains resident's right to privacy and dignity.

5. **Place clean linen on clean surface within reach (e.g., bedside stand, overbed table, or chair).**
   Prevents contamination of linen.

6. **Adjust bed to a safe working level, usually waist high. Lower head of bed before moving resident.**
   When bed is flat, resident can be moved without working against gravity.

7. **Put on gloves if linens are soiled with body fluids.**
   Prevents you from coming into contact with body fluids.

8. **Loosen top linen from the end of the bed or working side.**

9. **Raise side rail on far side of bed. After raising side rail, assist resident to turn onto side, moving away from you toward raised side rail (Fig. 6-47).**

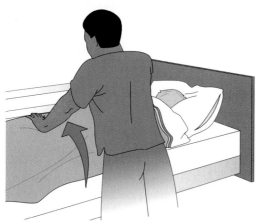

Fig. 6-47.

10. **Loosen bottom soiled linen on working side.**

11. **Roll bottom soiled linen toward resident tucking it snugly against resident's back.**
    Rolling puts dirtiest surface of linen inward, lessening contamination. The closer the linen is rolled to resident, the easier it is to remove from the other side.

12. **Place and tuck in clean bottom linen, finishing with bottom sheet free of wrinkles. Make hospital corners to keep bottom sheet wrinkle-free (Fig. 6-48).**
    Hospital corners prevent a resident's feet from

being restricted by or tangled in linen when getting in and out of bed.

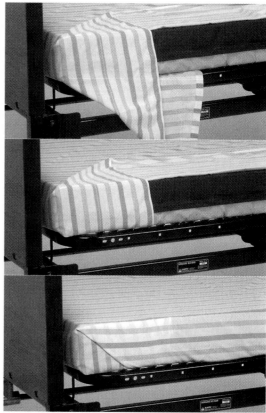

Fig. 6-48. Hospital corners help keep the sheet smooth under the resident.

13. **Assist resident to turn onto clean bottom sheet (Fig. 6-49). Raise side rail nearest you.**

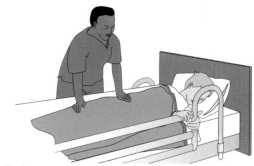

Fig. 6-49.

14. **Move to other side of bed and lower side rail.**

15. **Turn resident away from you toward side rail.**

16. **Loosen soiled linen. Roll linen from head to foot of bed. Avoid contact with your skin or clothes. Place it in a hamper/bag, at foot of the bed, or in a chair.**
    Always work from cleanest (head of bed) to dirtiest (foot of bed) to prevent spread of infection. Rolling puts dirtiest surface of linen inward, lessening contamination.

17. Pull and tuck in clean bottom linen, finishing with bottom sheet free of wrinkles (Fig. 6-50).

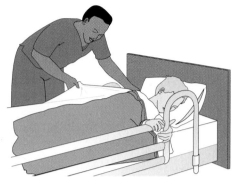

Fig. 6-50. Make hospital corners to keep bottom sheet wrinkle-free.

18. Place resident on his back. Raise side rail.

19. Remove pillow. Change pillowcase. (See box.) Place pillow under resident's head with open end away from door.

20. Cover resident with clean top sheet. Remove soiled top sheet.

21. Finish with the clean linen anchored and centered.

22. Unfold blanket over top sheet.

23. Tuck top linens under foot of mattress and make hospital corners.

24. Loosen top linens over resident's feet.
   Prevents pressure on feet, which can cause pressure sores.

25. Return bed to appropriate level. Put signaling device within resident's reach.
   Lowering the bed provides for safety. Signaling device allows resident to communicate with staff as necessary.

26. Dispose of soiled linen in the soiled linen container.

27. Remove gloves if worn.

28. Wash hands.
   Provides for infection control.

29. Report any changes in resident to the nurse.
   Provides nurse with information to assess resident.

30. Document procedure according to facility guidelines.
   What you write is a legal record of what you did. If you don't document it, legally it didn't happen.

Making an unoccupied bed

Equipment: clean linen: mattress pad, fitted or flat bottom sheet, waterproof bed protector if needed, blanket(s), cotton draw sheet, flat top sheet, pillowcase(s), gloves (if you're going to be touching linens soiled with body fluids)

1. Wash hands.
   Provides for infection control.

2. Place clean linen on clean surface within reach (e.g., bedside stand, overbed table, or chair).
   Prevents contamination of linen.

3. Adjust bed to a safe working level, usually waist high. Put bed in flattest position.
   Allows you to make a neat, wrinkle-free bed.

4. Put on gloves if linens are soiled with body fluids.
   Prevents you from coming into contact with body fluids.

5. Loosen soiled linen. Roll soiled linen (soiled side inside) from head to foot of bed. Avoid contact with your skin or clothes. Place it in a hamper/bag, at foot of the bed, or in chair.
   Always work from cleanest (head of bed) to dirtiest (foot of bed) to prevent spread of infection. Rolling puts dirtiest surface of linen inward, lessening risk of contamination.

6. Pull and tuck in clean bottom linen, finishing with bottom sheet free of wrinkles. Make hospital corners to keep bottom sheet wrinkle-free (Fig. 6-51, Fig. 6-52, Fig. 6-53).

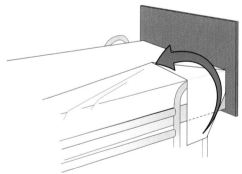

Fig. 6-51.

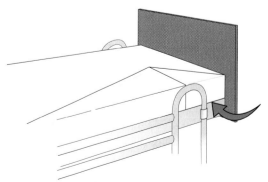

Fig. 6-52.

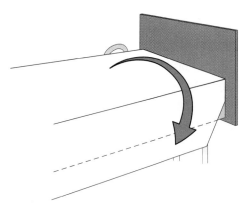

Fig. 6-53.

7. **Apply top linen. Finish with clean linen anchored and centered (Fig. 6-54).**

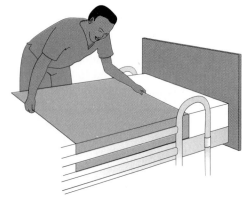

Fig. 6-54.

8. **Unfold blanket over top sheet.**

9. **Tuck top linens under foot of mattress and make hospital corners.**

10. **Replace pillowcase. (See box.) Place pillow under resident's head at head of the bed with open end away from door.**

11. **Return bed to appropriate level.**

12. **Dispose of soiled linen in the soiled linen container.**

13. **Remove gloves if worn.**

14. **Wash hands.**
    Provides for infection control.

A **closed bed** is a bed completely made with the bedspread and blankets in place. A closed bed is turned into an **open bed** by folding the linen down to the foot of the bed. Most residents are out of bed most of the day. A closed bed is made until it is time for the resident to go to sleep. Then an open bed is made.

Applying pillowcases

With one hand, grasp the clean pillowcase at the closed end. Turn it inside out over your arm. Next, using the same hand that has the pillowcase over it, grasp one narrow edge of the pillow. Pull the pillowcase over it with your free hand (Fig. 6-55).

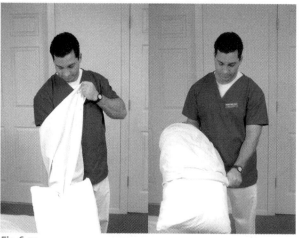

Fig. 6-55.

Unit 8: **Explain how to apply non-sterile dressings**

Sterile dressings are those that cover open or draining wounds. These dressings are always changed by a nurse. Non-sterile dressings are applied to dry wounds that have less chance of infection. Nursing assistants may assist with non-sterile dressing changes.

Changing a dry dressing using non-sterile technique

Equipment: package of square gauze dressings, adhesive tape, scissors, 2 pair of gloves

1. **Wash hands.**
   Provides for infection control.

2. **Identify yourself to resident by name. Address resident by name.**
   Resident has right to know identity of his or her caregiver. Addressing resident by name shows respect and establishes correct identification.

3. **Explain procedure to resident, speaking clearly, slowly, and directly, maintaining face-to-face contact whenever possible.**
   Promotes understanding and independence.

4. **Provide for resident's privacy during proce-**

dure with curtain, screen, or door.

Maintains resident's right to privacy and dignity.

5. Cut pieces of tape long enough to secure the dressing. Hang tape on the edge of a table within reach. Open four-inch gauze square package without touching gauze. Place the opened package on a flat surface.

6. Put on gloves.

    Protects you from coming into contact with body fluids.

7. Remove soiled dressing by gently peeling tape toward the wound. Lift dressing off the wound. Do not drag it over wound. Observe dressing for any odor. Notice color of the wound. Dispose of used dressing in proper container. Remove and dispose of gloves.

    Avoids disturbing wound healing. Reduces risk of contamination.

8. Put on new gloves. Touching only outer edges of new four-inch gauze, remove it from package. Apply it to wound. Tape gauze in place. Secure it firmly (Fig. 6-56).

    Keeps gauze as clean as possible.

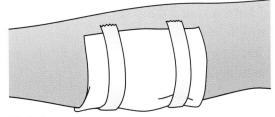

Fig. 6-56.

9. Remove and dispose of gloves properly.

10. Before leaving resident, place signaling device within resident's reach.

    Allows resident to communicate with staff as necessary.

11. Wash hands.

    Provides for infection control.

12. Report any changes in resident to the nurse.

    Provides nurse with information to assess resident.

13. Document procedure according to facility guidelines.

    What you write is a legal record of what you did. If you don't document it, legally it didn't happen.

SEVEN

Nutrition and Hydration

Unit 1: **Identify the six basic nutrients and the USDA Food Guide Pyramid**

Unit 2: **Demonstrate an awareness of regional, cultural, and religious food preferences**

Unit 3: **Explain special diets**

Unit 4: **Understand the importance of observing and reporting a resident's diet**

Unit 5: **Describe how to assist residents in maintaining fluid balance**

Unit 6: **List ways to identify and prevent unintended weight loss**

Unit 7: **Identify ways to promote appetites at mealtime**

Unit 8: **Demonstrate ways to feed residents**

Unit 9: **Describe eating and swallowing problems a resident may have**

Unit 1: Identify the six basic nutrients and the USDA Food Guide Pyramid

Good nutrition is very important. **Nutrition** is how the body uses food to maintain health. Our bodies need a well-balanced diet containing essential nutrients and plenty of fluids. This helps us grow new cells, maintain normal body function, and have energy for activities. Good nutrition in childhood and early adulthood helps ensure good health later in life. For those who are ill or elderly, a well-balanced diet helps maintain muscle and skin tissues and prevent pressure sores. A good diet also promotes the healing of wounds. It helps us cope with physical and emotional stress.

The Six Basic Nutrients

The body needs the following nutrients for growth and development:

1. **Protein.** Proteins are part of every body cell. They are essential for tissue growth and repair. Proteins are also an alternate supply of energy for the body.

Sources include fish, seafood, poultry, meat, eggs, milk, cheese, nuts, peas, and dried beans or legumes (Fig. 7-1).

Whole grain cereals, pastas, rice, and breads contain some proteins of lower quality. These must be complemented by a small quantity of the more complete proteins. Beans and rice or cereal and milk are examples of complementary proteins.

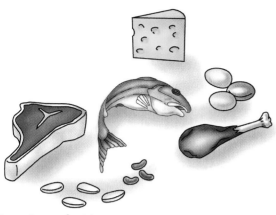

Fig. 7-1. Sources of protein.

2. **Carbohydrates**. Carbohydrates supply the fuel for the body's energy needs. They help the body use fat efficiently. Carbohydrates also provide fiber, which is necessary for bowel elimination.

Carbohydrates can be divided into two basic types: complex and simple carbohydrates. Complex carbohydrates are found in foods such as bread, cereal, potatoes, rice, pasta, vegetables, and fruits. Simple carbohydrates are found in foods such as sugars, sweets, syrups, and jellies. Simple carbohydrates do not have the same nutritional value as complex carbohydrates (Fig. 7-2).

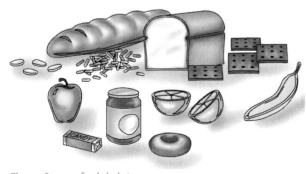

Fig. 7-2. Sources of carbohydrates.

The only value of simple carbohydrates is as a source of energy for people who eat very little or are malnourished. In other people, simple carbohydrates are stored as fat.

3. **Fats**. Fat helps the body store energy. Body fat also provides us with insulation. It protects body organs. In addition, fats are important for the absorption of certain vitamins.

Examples of fats are butter, margarine, salad dressings, oils, and animal fats found in meats, fowl, and fish (Fig. 7-3).

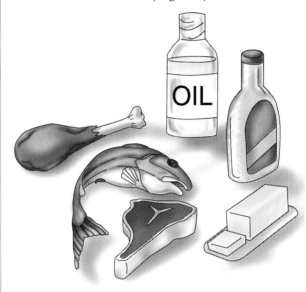

Fig. 7-3. Sources of fat.

Monounsaturated vegetable fats (including olive oil and canola oil) and polyunsaturated vegetable fats (including corn and safflower oils) are healthier kinds of fats. Saturated fats, including animal fats like butter, bacon and other fatty meats, are not as healthy. They should be limited in most diets.

♥ *Saturated fats raise the level of blood cholesterol. This can contribute to circulatory disorders.*

4. **Vitamins**. Vitamins are substances the body needs to function. The body cannot produce most vitamins. They can only be obtained from food, but they are essential to body functions. Vitamins A, D, E, and K are fat-soluble vitamins. This means they are carried and stored in body fat. Vitamins B and C are water-soluble vitamins that are broken down by water in our bodies. They cannot be stored in the body. They are eliminated in urine and feces.

Nutrition and Hydration

5. **Minerals**. Minerals form and maintain body cell functions. They provide energy and regulate processes. Zinc, iron, calcium, and magnesium are examples of minerals. Minerals are found in many foods.

6. **Water**. Because one-half to two-thirds of our body weight is water, we need about 6 to 8 glasses of water a day. Water is the most essential nutrient for life. Without it, a person can only live a few days. Water assists in the digestion and absorption of food. It helps with the elimination of waste. Through perspiration, water helps maintain normal body temperature. Maintaining enough fluid in our bodies is necessary for good health.

Most foods contain several nutrients, but no one food contains all the nutrients that are necessary to maintain a healthy body. Therefore, it is important to eat a daily diet that is well-balanced. Our diet should contain several foods selected from each of the food groups listed below.

The U.S. Department of Agriculture (USDA) has divided the foods that we eat into six groups:

1. Grains, including cereals, bread, rice, and pasta
2. Fruits
3. Vegetables
4. Dairy products
5. Meat, poultry, fish, eggs, dry beans, and nuts
6. Fats, oils, and sweets

These six groups have been arranged into the Food Guide Pyramid (Fig. 7-4). Foods close to the bottom of the pyramid should make up most of our diet. Foods closer to the top of the pyramid should be eaten in smaller quantities.

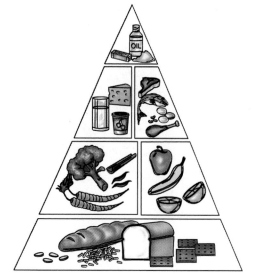

Fig. 7-4. The Food Guide Pyramid was created by the U.S. Department of Agriculture to show the six food groups. Together, they form a healthy diet.

Grains. Grains are found in cereal, bread, rice, and pasta. The Food Guide Pyramid recommends eating between six and eleven servings from the grain group each day. A **serving** is an individual portion or helping of food or drink. Grains are a great source of carbohydrates. Whole grain foods, such as whole wheat breads, bran cereals, brown rice, and whole wheat pastas contain more complex carbohydrates than white breads, rice, pastas, and processed cereals. They also contain more vitamins, protein, and energy.

Vegetables. Vegetables are excellent sources of vitamins and fiber. Choose from green leafy vegetables, including lettuce, spinach, and kale; tomatoes, green beans, peas, corn, cabbage, cauliflower, broccoli, and other vegetables. Vegetable sources of vitamin C include brussels sprouts, green or red peppers, and broccoli. The Food Guide Pyramid recommends eating three to five servings from the vegetable group each day. One serving from this group consists of ½ cup of cooked or chopped vegetables or ¾ cup of vegetable juice.

Fruits. Fruits are good sources of complex carbohydrates, vitamins, and fiber. Fruits are one of the best sources of vitamin C, a nutrient we should eat each day. Good sources of vitamin C include oranges and orange juice, grapefruit and grapefruit juice, strawberries, mango, papaya, and cantaloupe. The Food Guide Pyramid recommends eating two to four servings from the fruit group each day. One serving from this group could include one medium-sized apple, orange, banana, ¾ cup of juice, or ¼ cup of raisins.

Dairy Products. Milk and milk products, such as cheese and yogurt, are important sources of calcium. We need calcium for healthy bones and teeth. Milk products also contain other minerals, protein, and vitamins. Milk products include buttermilk, evaporated milk, and cottage cheese. Whole milk, cheese, and other products made with whole milk contain a lot of saturated fat. Most adults should eat low-fat or nonfat milk and milk products. Adults should have two to three servings from the dairy group each day. A serving is one cup of milk or yogurt, one-half cup of cottage cheese, or one-and-a-half ounces of cheese (Fig. 7-5).

Fish, Poultry, Meat, Eggs, Dry Beans, and Nuts. These foods provide protein, minerals, and vitamins. In addition, meat is a good source of iron. Lower-fat choices from this group include most fish, chicken or turkey breast, lean cuts of meat, and dry beans. The Food Guide Pyramid recommends eating two to three servings from this group each day. One serving from this group equals three ounces of cooked meat, one egg, ½ cup cooked dry beans, or ½ cup of nuts.

Fats, Oils, and Sweets. Fats and oils help the body absorb fat-soluble vitamins. They also provide flavor and make us feel full. Fats are needed by the body in very small quantities. Most adults eat more fat than their bodies need. Fats contain more than twice as many

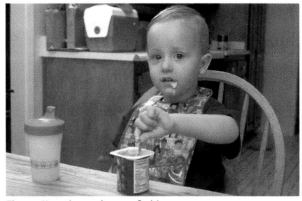

Fig. 7-5. Yogurt is a good source of calcium.

calories per gram as carbohydrates or proteins. Excess fat is stored by the body as fatty tissue. The best kinds of fats to use in a healthy diet are vegetable oils, including olive oil, canola oil, and corn oil. Sweets, including candy, cookies, cakes, pies, and ice cream, contain large quantities of fat and sugar. They should be eaten in much smaller quantities.

Unit 2: **Demonstrate an awareness of regional, cultural, and religious food preferences**

Culture, ethnicity, income, education, religion, and geography affect attitudes about nutrition. Food preferences may be formed by what you ate as a child, by what tastes good, or by personal beliefs about what should be eaten (Fig. 7-6). For instance, some people choose not to eat any animals or animal products, such as steak, chicken, butter, or eggs.

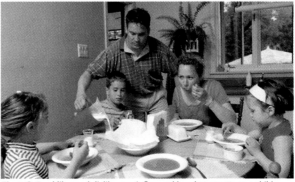

Fig. 7-6. Food likes and dislikes are influenced by what you ate as a child.

RA *Residents' rights include the right to make choices. This means that you must honor a resident's personal beliefs about selecting and avoiding specific foods.*

The region or culture you grew up in often influences your food preference. People from the southwestern United States may prefer spicy food. "Southern cooking" may include fried foods, like fried chicken or fried okra. Religious beliefs may influence diet too. For instance, some Muslim and Jewish people do not eat any pork.

Whatever your residents' food preference may be, respect it. Never make fun of a personal preference. If you notice that certain food is not being eaten—no matter how small the amount—report it to the nurse.

Unit 3: **Explain special diets**

A doctor sometimes places residents who have certain illnesses on modified diets. This diet is known as a **therapeutic**, or special, diet. Residents who do not eat enough may be placed on special supplementary diets. Diets are also prescribed for weight control and food allergies. Several types of modified diets are available for different types of illness, including the following:

Sodium-Restricted Diet (Low-Sodium Diet). Sodium is found in many foods, but people are most familiar with it as one of the two ingredients in table salt. Salt is the first food to be restricted in a low-sodium diet because it is high in sodium. Foods high in sodium include

- Cured meats: ham, bacon, lunch meat, sausage, salt pork, and hot dogs
- Salty or smoked fish: herring, salted cod, sardines, anchovies, caviar, smoked salmon or lox

- Processed cheese
- Canned and dried soups
- Vegetables preserved in brine: pickles, sauerkraut, olives, relishes
- Salted foods: nuts, dips, and spreads
- Sauces with high concentrations of salt: Worcestershire, barbecue, chili, and soy sauces
- Ketchup and mustard
- Canned foods
- Some cereals
- Over-the-counter medications and drugs (Fig. 7-7)

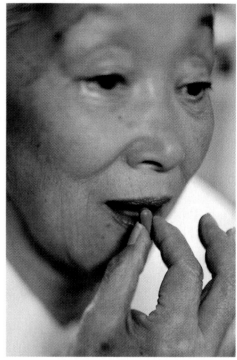

Fig. 7-7. Over-the-counter medications may be high in sodium.

Fluid-Restricted Diets. The amount of fluid taken into the body through food and fluids must equal the amount of fluid that leaves the body through perspiration, stool, urine, and expiration. This is **fluid balance**. When fluid intake is greater than fluid output, body tissue becomes swollen with excess fluid. In addition, people with severe heart disease or kidney disease may have difficulty processing large volumes of fluid. To prevent further heart or kidney damage, physicians may restrict a resident's fluid intake. For residents on fluid restriction, you will need to measure and document exact amounts of fluid intake and report excesses to the nurse.

Low-Protein Diet. In addition to restricted dietary intake of fluids and sodium, people who have kidney disease may also be on low-protein diets. Protein is restricted because it breaks down into compounds that may lead to further kidney damage. The extent of the restrictions depends on the stage of the disease and whether the resident is on dialysis.

Low-Fat/Low-Cholesterol Diet. People who have high levels of cholesterol in their blood are at risk for heart attacks and heart disease. People with gallbladder disease, diseases that interfere with fat digestion, and liver disease are also placed on low-fat/low-cholesterol diets. Low-fat/low-cholesterol diets permit skim milk, low-fat cottage cheese, fish, white meat of turkey and chicken, veal, and vegetable fats (especially monounsaturated fats such as olive, canola, and peanut oils) (Fig. 7-8). Residents may be advised to limit their diets in the following ways:

- Eat lean cuts of meat including lamb, beef, and pork, and limit even these to three times a week.

- Limit egg yolks to three or four per week (including eggs used in baking).

- Avoid organ meats, shellfish, fatty meats, cream, butter, lard, meat drippings, coconut and palm oils, and desserts and soups made with whole milk.

- Avoid fried foods and sweets.

People who have gallbladder disease or other digestive problems may be placed on a diet that restricts all fats.

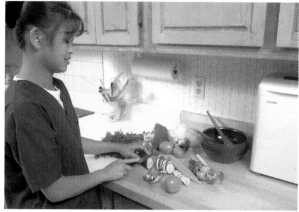

Fig. 7-8. Eating plenty of fresh vegetables is an important part of a low-fat diet.

Modified Calorie Diet for Weight Management. Some residents may need to reduce calories to lose weight or prevent additional weight gain. Other residents may need to gain weight or increase calories because of malnutrition, surgery, illness, or fever. Residents with certain conditions need more protein to promote growth and repair of tissue and regulation of body functions.

Dietary Management of Ulcers. Ulcers can be irritated by foods that produce or increase levels of acid in the stomach. People who have ulcers usually know the foods that cause them discomfort. Physicians will advise them to avoid these foods, as well as the following: alcohol; beverages containing caffeine, such as coffee, tea, and soft drinks; and spicy seasonings such as black pepper, cayenne, and chili pepper. Three meals or more a day are usually advised. If alcohol is allowed, it should be consumed with meals.

Dietary Management of Diabetes Mellitus. Calories and carbohydrates are carefully regulated in the dietary management of diabetic residents (see Chapter 8 for more information on this disorder). Protein and fats are also regulated. The types of foods and the amounts are determined by the resident's nutritional and energy requirements. Two types of diets can manage diabetes mellitus:

1. **Non-Concentrated Sweets Diet**. This diet is a regular, well-balanced diet that excludes concentrated sweets, such as sugars, honey, syrup, jellies, jams, preserves, candy, and cranberry sauce. The diet also eliminates cakes, pastries, cookies, puddings, ice cream, gelatin, sweetened fruit juices and beverages, sugar-coated cereals, condensed milk, and candied or glazed fruits and vegetables.

2. **Exchange List Diets**. This type of diet involves more than just the elimination of concentrated sweets. Meals are carefully planned based on exact amounts of food from the six food groups. Exchange lists are then used to determine foods and the exact serving sizes that may be eaten to follow the meal plan. Foods are measured and must be eaten completely at certain times. Eating the necessary carbohydrates, which are found in dairy and bread groups, is very important if the resident is too ill to tolerate the other foods. Any variation in eating patterns and routine must be reported to the nurse.

♥ *Understanding the effects of certain illnesses and diseases on the body helps you realize the reasons for special diets.*

Unit 4: Understand the importance of observing and reporting a resident's diet

Help residents on their special diets by checking their trays or plates to make sure all the foods are permitted. Mistakes may happen in the kitchen. Before delivering trays or plates, check them closely. Make sure that you have the correct resident and the correct food and beverages for that resident. Trays should also be closely checked for added sugar and salt packets. Always check diet trays for dentures, glasses, and hearing aides before removing them.

Some residents eat in dining rooms. It is just as important to observe the food being served there (Fig. 7-9). Be aware of residents who are diabetic or have heart conditions. They will be on special diets. Their families may not know or understand about food restrictions. Family often brings treats into the facility for their loved ones. Watch for foods in residents' rooms that are not permitted by their doctors. Report any problems to the nurse.

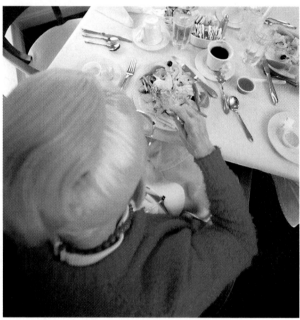

Fig. 7-9. Observe residents' plates for any restricted food.

Two common food errors for elderly residents on special diets are

1. Residents eat too much salt and sodium by adding salt at the table. Or they unknowingly choose foods high in sodium.

2. Residents eat too many concentrated sweets without realizing how high the sugar content is.

Food trays and plates should also be observed after the resident completes the meal. It is important for the staff to observe what and how much the resident is eating. This helps to identify residents with poor appetites. It may also signal a problem such as dentures that do not fit properly or are in bad condition.

Facilities keep track of the amount of food and liquid a resident consumes. This method varies from one facility to another. Some facilities use a percentage method to record food intake. Below is one example of a percentage method.

- "R" Refused = 0% No food eaten
- "P" Poor = 25% Very little food eaten
- "F" Fair = 50% Half of the food eaten
- "G" Good = 75% Most of the food is eaten
- "A" All = 100% Entire meal is eaten

Other facilities may document the percentage of specific foods eaten—protein, carbohydrates, fats, etc. It is important for you to follow facility policy. Document food intake very carefully.

Unit 5: **Describe how to assist residents in maintaining fluid balance**

Most residents should be encouraged to drink six to eight glasses of water a day. Remember, water is an essential nutrient for life. The sense of thirst can diminish as people age. Remind your elderly residents to drink fluids often (Fig. 7-10). However, some residents will have an order to force fluids (FF) or restrict fluids (RF) because of medical conditions. Make sure you know which residents have these special orders.

Dehydration occurs when a person does not have enough fluid in the body. Dehydration is a major problem among the elderly, in and out of nursing homes. People can become dehydrated if they do not drink enough or if they have diarrhea or are vomiting.

OBSERVING AND REPORTING
Dehydration

Report any of the following immediately:

- resident drinks less than six 8oz glasses of liquid per day

- resident needs help drinking from a cup or glass
- resident has trouble swallowing liquids
- resident experiences frequent vomiting, diarrhea, or fever
- resident is easily confused or tired

resident has one or more of the following:

- dry mouth
- cracked lips
- sunken eyes
- dark urine
- strong-smelling urine

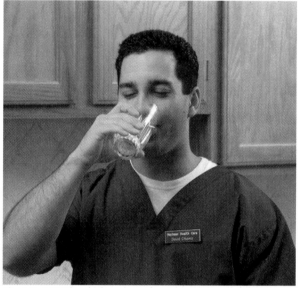

Fig. 7-10. Remember, drinking plenty of water is good for you, too!

GUIDELINES
Preventing Dehydration

- Report observations and warning signs to the nurse immediately.
- Encourage residents to drink every time you see them (Fig. 7-11).
- Offer fresh water or other fluids often.
- Record fluid intake and output.
- Ice chips, frozen flavored ice sticks, and gelatin are also forms of liquids. Offer them often. Do not offer ice chips or sticks if a resident has a swallowing problem.

Ⓖ If appropriate, offer sips of liquid between bites of food at meals and snacks.

Ⓖ Make sure pitcher and cup are near
enough and light enough for the resident to lift.

Ⓖ Offer the appropriate assistance if resident cannot drink without help.

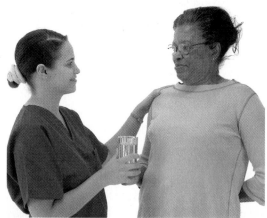

Fig. 7-11. Encouraging residents to drink every time you see them can help prevent dehydration.

Serving fresh water

Equipment: water pitcher, ice scoop, glass, straw

1. **Wash hands.**
    Provides for infection control.

2. **Identify yourself to resident by name.
    Address resident by name.**
    *Resident has right to know identity of his or her
    caregiver. Addressing resident by name shows re-
    spect and establishes correct identification.*

3. **Scoop ice into water pitcher. Add fresh
    water.**

4. **Use and store ice scoop properly:**

    **Do not allow ice to touch hand and fall back
    into container.**

    **Place scoop in appropriate receptacle after
    each use.**
    Avoids contamination of ice.

5. **Take pitcher of ice water to resident.**

6. **Pour glass of water for resident and leave
    pitcher and glass at the bedside.**
    Encourages resident to maintain hydration.

7. **Make sure that pitcher and glass are light
    enough for resident to lift. Leave a straw if
    the resident desires.**
    *Demonstrates understanding of resident's abilities
    and/or limitations. Prevents dehydration.*

8. **Before leaving resident, place signaling**

device within resident's reach.
*Allows resident to communicate with staff as neces-
sary.*

9. **Wash hands.**
    Provides for infection control.

👁 *You must be very careful not to contaminate the ice each time you scoop it. Never
touch the ice and allow it to fall back into the
container. Make sure the scoop is placed in
the proper place after each use.*

Fluid overload occurs when the body is unable to handle the amount of fluid consumed. This condition often affects people
with heart or kidney disease.

OBSERVING AND REPORTING
Fluid Overload

Ⓞ swelling/edema of extremities (ankles,
feet, fingers, hands)

Ⓞ weight gain (daily weight gain of one to
two pounds)

Ⓞ decreased urine output

Ⓞ shortness of breath

Ⓞ increased heart rate

Ⓞ skin that appears tight, smooth, and
shiny

Unit 6: List ways to identify and prevent unintended weight loss

Just like dehydration, unintended weight
loss is a big problem for the elderly. Weight
loss can mean that the resident has a serious
medical condition. It can lead to skin breakdown, which leads to pressure sores. It is
very important to report any weight loss you
notice, no matter how small (Fig. 7-12). If a
resident has diabetes, chronic obstructive
pulmonary disease, cancer, HIV, or other diseases, he is at a greater risk for malnutrition.
(See chapter 8 for more information on
these diseases.)

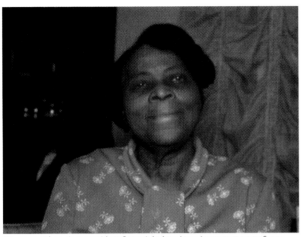

Fig. 7-12. Observing a resident for weight loss is an important part of your job.

OBSERVING AND REPORTING
Unintended Weight Loss:

Report any of the following immediately:

- resident needs help eating or drinking
- resident eats less than half of meals/snacks served
- resident has mouth pain
- resident has dentures that do not fit properly
- resident has difficulty chewing or swallowing
- resident coughs or chokes while eating
- resident is sad, has crying spells, or withdraws from others
- resident is confused, wanders, or paces

GUIDELINES
Preventing Unintended Weight Loss

- Report observations and warning signs to the nurse.
- Encourage residents to eat.
- Honor food likes and dislikes.
- Offer many different kinds of foods and beverages.
- Help residents who have trouble feeding themselves.
- Allow enough time to finish eating.

- Notify nurse if resident has trouble using utensils.
- Record meal/snack intake.
- Provide oral care before and after meals.
- Position residents sitting upright for feeding.
- If resident has had a loss of appetite and/or seems sad, ask about it.

Regulations require that the intake of food and fluids be monitored to prevent malnutrition and dehydration. Nursing assistants have a responsibility to assist residents with eating and drinking so that they are nourished and hydrated.

Unit 7: Identify ways to promote appetites at mealtime

Mealtime is an important part of a resident's day. This is especially true because weight loss and malnutrition issues are common among the elderly. Illness, pain, and medications may cause loss of appetite. To encourage healthy eating, do all that you can to promote a resident's appetite. Mealtime should be made as pleasant as possible.

GUIDELINES
Promoting Appetites

- Offer a trip to the bathroom or assist with toileting before eating.
- Assist residents with handwashing before the meal arrives.
- Provide oral care before eating.
- Assists resident to comfortable position.
- Serve food at the correct temperature.
- Plates and trays should look appetizing.
- Provide the resident with the proper eating tools. Use adaptive utensils if needed. (See chapter 9.)
- Be social and friendly during mealtime.

Nutrition and Hydration

Talk with residents if they wish to do so (Fig. 7-13).

Ⓖ Provide additional food when requested.

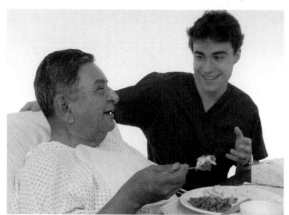

Fig. 7-13. Be pleasant and friendly while residents are eating.

Unit 8: Demonstrate ways to feed residents

One important nursing assistant duty is assisting residents with their meals. Some residents will be unable to feed themselves. It will be your responsibility to feed them. Residents who must be fed are often embarrassed and depressed about their dependence on another person. Be aware of this. Provide plenty of privacy while the resident is eating. Do not rush the person. Encourage residents to do whatever they can for themselves. For example, if a resident can hold and use a napkin, she should. If she can hold and eat finger foods, offer them. There are special devices that can assist residents with eating. Cups with lids to avoid spills and utensils with thick handles that are easier to hold are two examples. More adaptive devices are shown in chapter 9.

Rℐ *If a resident does not want to use a clothing protector while eating, that is his or her right. Respect the resident's wishes.*

GUIDELINES
Assisting a Resident with Eating

Ⓖ Never treat the resident like a child. This is embarrassing and disrespectful. It is difficult for many people to accept help with feeding. Be as supportive and encouraging as you can.

Ⓖ Sit at a resident's eye level.

Ⓖ Check the temperature at your wrist before offering a bite of food.

Ⓖ Cut foods and pour liquids as needed.

Ⓖ Ask the resident which food he prefers to eat first. Allow him to make the choice, even if he wants to eat dessert first.

Ⓖ Do not rush the meal. Appear relaxed.

Ⓖ Make simple conversation. Try not to ask questions that require answers.

Ⓖ Give the resident your full attention during eating.

Ⓖ Alternate offering food and drink.

Before feeding or assisting with feeding, prepare the food by following these steps. Only do what the resident is unable to do for himself.

C: *Cut meat, vegetables, etc.*

O: *Open milk carton and put in straw.*

B: *Butter roll, bread, or vegetables.*

S: *Season food the way resident prefers.*

Feeding a resident who cannot feed self

Equipment: meal tray, clothing protector, 1-2 washcloths

1. **Wash hands.**
   Provides for infection control.

2. **Identify yourself to resident by name. Address resident by name.**
   Resident has right to know identity of his or her caregiver. Addressing resident by name shows respect and establishes correct identification.

3. **Explain procedure to resident, speaking clearly, slowly, and directly, maintaining face-to-face contact whenever possible.**
   Promotes understanding and independence

4. **Assist resident to wash hands.**
   Promotes good hygiene and infection control.

5. **Before feeding resident, ensure resident is in an upright sitting position (at a 90 degree angle) (Fig. 7-14).**
Promotes ease of swallowing. Prevents aspiration of food and beverage.

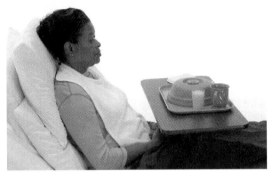

Fig. 7-14.

6. **Pick up name card. Verify that resident has received the tray prepared for him/her.**
Tray should only contain foods, fluids, and condiments permitted on the diet.

7. **Assist resident to put on clothing protector, if desired.**
Protects resident's clothing from food and beverage spills.

8. **Sit at resident's eye level (Fig. 7-15).**
Promotes good communication. Lets resident know that he or she will not be rushed while eating.

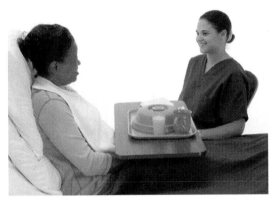

Fig. 7-15.

9. **Offer drink of beverage. Alternate types of food offered, allowing for resident's preferences. (Do not feed all of one type before offering another type.)**
Resident has right to make decisions.

10. **Offer the food in bite-sized pieces. Report any swallowing difficulties to the nurse immediately (Fig. 7-16).**
Small pieces are easier to chew. Lessens risk of choking.

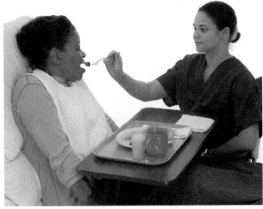

Fig. 7-16.

11. **Make sure resident's mouth is empty before next bite of food or sip of beverage.**
Lessens risk of choking.

12. **Offer beverage to resident throughout the meal.**
Promotes ease of swallowing.

13. **Talk with resident during meal.**
Makes mealtime more enjoyable.

14. **Wipe food from resident's mouth and hands as necessary during the meal. Wipe again at the end of the meal (Fig. 7-17).**
Maintains resident's dignity.

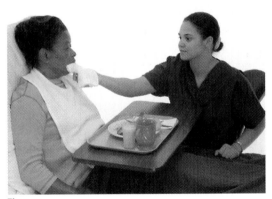

Fig. 7-17.

15. **Remove clothing protector if used. Dispose of in proper container.**

16. **Before leaving resident, place signaling device within resident's reach.**
Allows resident to communicate with staff as necessary.

17. **Remove food tray. Check for eyeglasses, dentures, or any personal items.**

18. **Wash hands.**
Provides for infection control.

19. **Report any changes in resident to the nurse.**
Provides nurse with information to assess resident.

Nutrition and Hydration

20. **Document procedure according to facility guidelines.**

    What you write is a legal record of what you did. If you don't document it, legally it didn't happen.

☝ *You must offer fluid to the resident throughout the meal. You must also remember to raise the head of the bed to help prevent aspiration.*

Unit 9: Describe eating and swallowing problems a resident may have

Residents may have conditions that make eating or swallowing difficult. A stroke, or CVA, can cause weakness on one side of the body and paralysis. Nerve and muscle damage from head and neck cancer, multiple sclerosis, Parkinson's or Alzheimer's disease may be present. You will learn more about these diseases in chapter 8. If a resident has difficulty swallowing, soft foods and thickened liquids will be served. A straw or special cup will help make swallowing easier.

Swallowing problems put residents at high risk for choking on food or drink. Inhaling food or drink into the lungs is called **aspiration**. Aspiration can cause pneumonia or death. Alert the nurse immediately if any problems occur while feeding the resident.

GUIDELINES
Preventing Aspiration

- Position resident properly. They must sit in a straight, upright position. Do not try to feed a resident in a reclining position.

- Offer small pieces of food or small spoons of pureed food.

- Feed resident slowly.

- Place food in the non-paralyzed or unaffected side of the mouth.

- Make sure mouth is empty before next bite of food or sip of drink.

When a person is completely unable to swallow, he or she may be fed through a special tube. A **nasogastric tube** is inserted into the nose going to the stomach. A **gastrostomy tube** is inserted through the abdomen, into the stomach. (More information on care of gastric tubes is in chapter 6.) If a person's digestive system does not function properly, **hyperalimentation** or **total parenteral nutrition (TPN)** may be necessary. With TPN a resident receives nutrients directly into the bloodstream. It bypasses the digestive system.

With all of these different types of feeding, make sure that the tubing is not kinked or pulled in any way.

EIGHT

Common, Chronic, and Acute Conditions

Residents in long-term care may have many different diseases and conditions. Diseases and conditions are considered acute or chronic. **Acute** means an illness has severe symptoms. An acute illness is short-term. **Chronic** means the disease or condition is long-term or long-lasting. However, symptoms are managed. Chronic conditions are usually less severe from day to day. Chronic conditions may have short periods of severity. During this time, the person may be hospitalized to stabilize the disease. This book discusses diseases or conditions according to the body system in which they are classified.

The following is a partial list of the body systems you learned in chapter 4:

- Musculoskeletal
- Nervous
- Circulatory or cardiovascular
- Respiratory
- Urinary
- Gastrointestinal or digestive
- Endocrine
- Reproductive
- Immune and Lymphatic

Common, Chronic, and Acute Conditions

If you think of the body system under which a disease is classified, the signs and symptoms will be easier to remember. In this chapter, we list only the most common diseases and conditions in long-term care. Information on pressure sores, which are a common disorder of the integumentary system, is in chapter 5.

Unit 1: Describe common diseases and disorders of the musculoskeletal system

Arthritis

Arthritis is a general term that refers to **inflammation**, or swelling, of the joints. It causes stiffness, pain, and decreased mobility. Arthritis may be the result of aging, injury, or an **autoimmune illness**. With an autoimmune illness, the body's immune system attacks normal tissue in the body. There are several types of arthritis.

1. **Osteoarthritis**. Osteoarthritis is a common type of arthritis that affects the elderly. It may occur with aging or as the result of joint injury. Hips and knees, which are weight-bearing joints, are usually affected. Joints of the fingers, thumbs, and spine can also be affected. Pain and stiffness seem to increase in cold or damp weather.

2. **Rheumatoid Arthritis**. Rheumatoid arthritis can affect people of all ages. Joints become inflamed, red, swollen, and very painful. Movement is eventually restricted. Fever, fatigue, and weight loss are also symptoms (Fig. 8-1).

Arthritis is generally treated with some or all of the following:

- anti-inflammatory medications such as aspirin or ibuprofen

- local applications of heat to reduce swelling and pain

- range of motion exercises (Chapter 9)

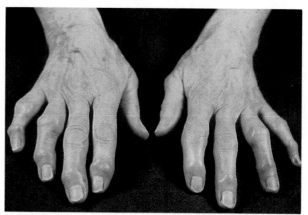

Fig. 8-1. Rheumatoid arthritis. (Photo courtesy Frederick Miller, MD.)

- regular exercise and/or activity routines

- diet to reduce weight or maintain strength

GUIDELINES
Caring for Residents with Arthritis

- Watch for stomach irritation or heartburn caused by aspirin or ibuprofen. Some residents cannot take these medications. Report signs of stomach irritation immediately.

- Encourage activity. Gentle activity can help reduce the effects of arthritis. Follow care plan instructions carefully. Use canes or other walking aids as needed.

- Adapt activities of daily living (ADLs) to allow independence. Many devices are available to allow residents to bathe, dress, and feed themselves even when they have arthritis. (See chapter 9.)

- Choose clothing that is easy to put on and fasten. Encourage use of handrails and safety bars in the bathroom.

- Treat each resident as an individual. Arthritis is very common among elderly residents. Do not assume that each resident has the same symptoms and needs the same care.

- Help resident's self-esteem by encouraging self-care. Maintain a positive attitude. Listen to the resident's feelings.

Osteoporosis

Osteoporosis is a disease that causes bones to become brittle. Brittle bones can break easily. Weakness in the bones may be due to age, lack of hormones, not enough calcium in bones, alcohol consumption, or lack of exercise. Nursing assistants must move and reposition residents with osteoporosis very carefully.

Osteoporosis occurs more commonly in women after menopause. **Menopause** is the stopping of menstrual periods. Extra calcium and regular exercise can help prevent osteoporosis. Medication, calcium, and fluoride supplements are used to treat osteoporosis.

Signs and symptoms of osteoporosis include

- low back pain
- loss of height
- stooped posture (Fig. 8-2)

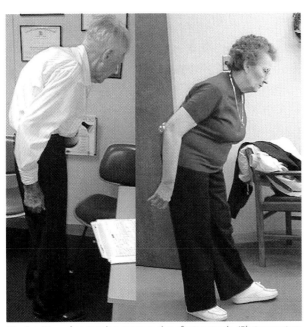

Fig. 8-2. Stooped posture is a common sign of osteoporosis. (Photos courtesy of Jeffrey T. Behr, MD.)

Fractures and Hip/Knee Replacement

A **fracture** is a broken bone. Fractures are usually due to weakened bones. Preventing falls, which can lead to fractures, is very important. Fractures of arms, elbows, legs, and hips are the most common.

Total hip replacement is surgery that replaces the head of the long bone of the leg (femur) where it joins the hip. This is done for any of the following reasons:

- Fractured hip due to an injury or fall which does not heal properly (Fig. 8-3)

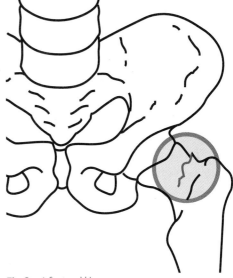

Fig. 8-3. A fractured hip.

- Weakened hip due to aging
- Hip that is painful and stiff because the joint is weak and the bones are no longer strong enough to bear the weight of the person

The surgery is done through a cut at the hip. An artificial ball and socket joint replaces the hip. After the surgery, the resident is not able to stand on that leg while the hip heals. A physical therapist will assist after surgery. The goals of care include slowly strengthening the hip muscles and getting the resident walking on that leg.

As always, be familiar with the resident's care plan. It will state when the resident may begin putting weight on the hip. It will also tell how much the resident is permitted to do. It is important to assist with personal care and using assistive devices, such as walkers or canes.

GUIDELINES
Caring for Residents Recovering from Hip Replacements

Ⓖ Keep often-used items, such as medications, telephone, tissues, call light, and water within easy reach. Avoid placing items needed by the resident in high places.

Ⓖ Dress starting with the affected side first.

Ⓖ Never rush the resident. Use praise and encouragement.

Ⓖ Have the resident sit to do tasks and save energy.

Ⓖ Follow the care plan exactly, even if the resident wants to do more than is ordered.

Ⓖ Never perform ROM exercises on a leg on the side of a hip replacement unless directed by the nurse.

Ⓖ Caution the resident not to sit with legs crossed. The hip cannot be at less than a 90-degree angle. It cannot be turned outward (Fig. 8-4).

OBSERVING AND REPORTING
Hip Replacement

◉ incision is red, draining, or warm to touch

◉ an increase in pain

◉ abnormal vital signs, especially elevated temperature

◉ ability to use equipment properly and safely

◉ following doctor's orders for activity and exercise

◉ appetite and nutrition management

◉ increasing strength and improving ability to walk

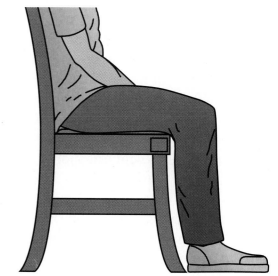

Fig. 8-4. The hip must maintain a 90-degree angle in the sitting position.

Total knee replacement is the surgical insertion of a prosthetic knee. This is performed to relieve pain. It also restores motion to a knee damaged by injury or arthritis. Care is similar to that for the hip replacement. However, the recovery time is much shorter. These residents have more ability to care for themselves.

Unit 2: Describe common diseases and disorders of the nervous system

Dementia

As we age, we may lose some of our ability to think logically and quickly. This ability is called **cognition**. When we lose some of this ability, we are said to have cognitive impairment. Cognitive impairment affects concentration and memory. Elderly residents may lose their memories of recent events, which can be frustrating for them. You can help by encouraging them to make lists of things to remember and writing down names and phone numbers.

Other normal changes of aging in the brain include slower reaction time, difficulty finding or using the right words, and sleeping less.

Dementia is a more serious loss of mental abilities such as thinking, remembering, reasoning, and communicating. As dementia advances, these losses make it difficult to perform ADLs such as eating, bathing, dressing, and toileting. **Dementia is not a normal part of aging**.

The following are some of the causes of dementia:

- Alzheimer's disease
- Multi-infarct dementia (a series of strokes causing damage to the brain)
- Parkinson's disease
- Huntington's disease
- AIDS
- metabolic imbalances
- circulatory disorders

Alzheimer's Disease (AD)

Alzheimer's disease causes tangled nerve fibers and protein deposits to form in the brain, eventually causing dementia. The disease gets worse, causing greater and greater loss of health and abilities. The disease cannot be cured. Residents with AD will never recover. They will need more care as the disease progresses.

AD generally begins with forgetfulness and confusion. It progresses to complete loss of all ability to care for oneself. Each person with AD will show different symptoms at different times. For example, one person with Alzheimer's may be able to read, but not use the phone or remember her own address. Another person with Alzheimer's may have lost the ability to read, but may still be able to do simple math. Skills a person has used constantly over a long lifetime are usually kept longer.

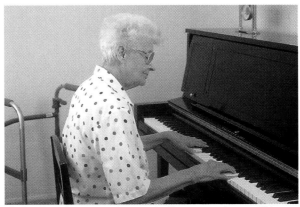

Fig. 8-5. Even when a person loses much of her memory, she may still keep skills she has used her whole life.

Encourage residents with AD to perform ADLs and keep their minds and bodies as active as possible. Working, socializing, reading, problem solving, and exercising should all be encouraged (Fig. 8-6). Having residents with AD do as much as possible for themselves may even help slow the progression of the disease. Look for tasks that are challenging but not frustrating. Help your residents succeed in performing them.

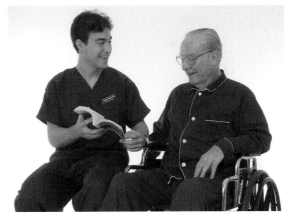

Fig. 8-6. Encourage reading and thinking activities for residents with AD.

GUIDELINES
Working with Residents with AD

- Do not take their behavior personally.
- Treat residents with AD with dignity and respect, as you would want to be treated.
- Work with the symptoms and behaviors you see.

Common, Chronic, and Acute Conditions

- Work as a team.
- Encourage communication.
- Take care of yourself.
- Work with family members.
- Follow the goals of the resident care plan.

GUIDELINES
Communicating with Residents who have AD

- Speak in a low, calm voice, in a room that has very little background noise and distraction.
- Repeat yourself, using the same words and phrases, as often as needed.
- Use pictures or use gestures to help communicate.
- Break complex tasks into simple tasks.

Use the same procedures for personal care for residents with AD. However, there are some guidelines to keep in mind when assisting these residents. Three general principles will help you give your residents the best care:

1. Develop a routine and stick to it. Being consistent is very important when working with residents who are confused and easily upset.

2. Promote self-care. Help your residents to care for themselves as much as possible. This will help them cope with this difficult disease.

3. Take good care of yourself, both mentally and physically. This will help you give the best care.

GUIDELINES
Caring for Residents with AD

- Ensure safety by using nonslip mats, tub seats, and hand holds.

- Schedule bathing when the resident is least upset. Be organized so the bath can be quick.
- Always use the same steps, explaining in the same way every time.
- Assist with grooming. Help the people in your care feel attractive and dignified.
- Set up a regular schedule for toileting and follow it.
- Mark the restroom with a sign or a picture as a reminder to use it and where it is.
- Maintain a daily exercise routine.
- Maintain the best nutrition.
- Maintain self-esteem by encouraging independence in ADLs.
- Share in enjoyable activities, looking at pictures, and talking.
- Reward positive and independent behavior with smiles, hugs, warm touches, and thank yous (Fig. 8-7).

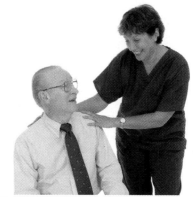

Fig. 8-7. Reward positive behavior with warm touches, smiles, and thank yous.

- Try to identify the causes or "triggers" of agitated behavior and remove them.

Below are some common difficult behaviors that you may face when working with Alzheimer's residents:

- **Agitation.** Try to remove triggers. Keep routine constant. Avoid frustration. Help resident focus on a soothing, familiar activity, such as sorting things or looking at pictures. Remain calm and use a low, soothing voice to speak to and reassure the resident. An arm around the shoulder, patting gently, or lightly stroking may be soothing for some residents.

- **Pacing and Wandering**. A resident who walks back and forth in the same area is pacing. A resident who walks aimlessly around the nursing home is wandering. Restlessness, hunger, disorientation, need for toileting, constipation, pain, forgetting how or where to sit down, or too much daytime napping may cause pacing and wandering (Fig. 8-8).

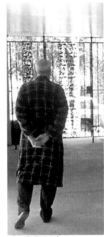

Fig. 8-8. Make sure a resident is in a safe area if he paces or wanders.

- **Hallucinations or Delusions**. A resident who sees things that are not there is having hallucinations. A resident who believes things that are not true is having delusions. Reassure a resident who seems agitated or worried. Do not argue with a resident who is imagining things. Do not tease or make fun of the resident. Be calm. Reassure resident that you are there to help. Do not tell the resident that the delusion is true.

- **Sundowning**. When a person becomes restless and agitated in the late afternoon, evening, or night, it is called sundowning. Remove triggers. Provide snacks or encourage rest. Avoid stressful situations during this time. Limit activities, appointments, trips, and visits. Play soft music. Set a bedtime routine and keep it. Recognize when sundowning occurs and plan a calming activity just before. Eliminate caffeine from the diet. Give a soothing back massage. Distract the resident with a simple, calm activity like looking at a magazine.

- **Perseveration or Repetitive Phrasing**. A resident who repeats a word, phrase, question, or activity over and over is **perseverating**. Respond to this with patience. Do not try to silence or stop the resident. Answer questions each time they are asked, using the same words each time.

- **Violent Behavior**. A resident who attacks, hits, or threatens someone is violent. Frustration or overstimulation may trigger violence. It can also be triggered by a change in routine, environment, or caregiver. Look for ways to avoid these triggers. Report any extreme or unusual behavior to the nurse.

The following are appropriate responses to violent residents:

- Block blows but never hit back (Fig. 8-9).

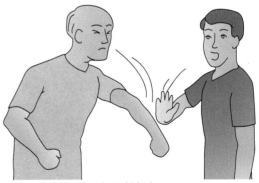

Fig. 8-9. Block blows but do not hit back.

- Step out of reach.

- Call for help if needed.

- Try to remove triggers. If you are the trigger, step outside to seek help. A resident may respond better to another staff member.

Although AD cannot be cured, there are many techniques that can improve the quality of life for residents with AD.

Reality orientation is using calendars, clocks, signs, and lists to help residents remember who and where they are. In later stages of AD, reality orientation may only frustrate residents. It useful in the early stages of AD when residents are confused but not totally disoriented.

Validation therapy means letting residents believe they live in the past or in imaginary circumstances. Do not argue with or correct them. Instead, explore the resident's beliefs. **Validating** means giving value to or approving. Make no attempt to reorient the resident to actual circumstances, which can agitate them. Validating can provide comfort and reduce agitation. It is useful in cases of moderate to severe disorientation.

Reminiscence therapy is encouraging residents to remember and talk about the past. Explore memories by asking about details (Fig. 8-10). Focus on a time of life that was pleasant. Work through feelings about a difficult time in the past. It is useful in many stages of AD, but especially with moderate to severe confusion.

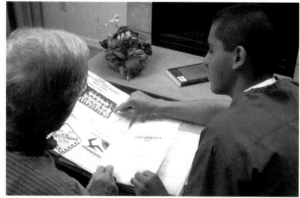

Fig. 8-10. Reminiscence therapy is encouraging a resident to remember and talk about the past.

Activity therapy uses activities residents enjoy to prevent boredom and frustration. They also promote self-esteem. Helping your resident to take walks, do puzzles, listen to music, read, or do other activities she enjoys is useful throughout most stages of AD.

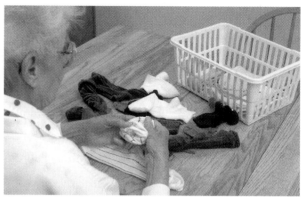

Fig. 8-11. Activities that are not frustrating can be helpful for residents with AD. They promote mental exercise.

Parkinson's Disease

Parkinson's disease is a progressive disease. It causes a section of the brain to degenerate. It affects the muscles, causing them to become stiff. In addition, it causes stooped posture and a shuffling **gait**, or walk. Tremors or shaking make it very difficult for a person to do ADLs such as eating and bathing. A person with Parkinson's may have a mask-like facial expression.

Medications may help. Residents are at a high risk for falls. Encourage self-care. Protect residents from any unsafe areas and conditions.

Multiple Sclerosis (MS)

When a person has MS, the protective covering for the nerves, spinal cord, and white matter of the brain breaks down over time. Without this covering, or sheath, nerves cannot send messages to and from the brain in a normal way. Signs and symptoms include blurred vision, tremors, poor balance, and difficulty walking. Weakness, numbness, tingling, incontinence, and behavior changes are also symptoms. Residents with MS can eventually develop blindness, contractures (see chapter 9), and loss of function in the arms and legs.

Be patient with self-care and movement. Allow the resident enough time to do things.

Prevent falls, which may be due to a lack of coordination, fatigue, and vision problems.

CVA or Stroke

The medical term for a stroke is a cerebrovascular accident (CVA). It is caused when blood supply to a part of the brain is cut off suddenly by a clot or a ruptured blood vessel (Fig. 8-12). Without blood, part of the brain gets no oxygen. This causes the brain cells to die. See chapter 2 for more information on the warning signs of a stroke.

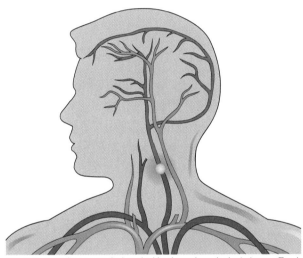

Fig. 8-12. A stroke is caused when the blood supply to the brain is cut off suddenly by a clot or ruptured blood vessel.

The two sides of the brain control different things. Symptoms depend on which side of the brain the stroke affected. Weaknesses on the right side of the body show that the left side of the brain was affected. Weaknesses on the left side of the body show that the right side of the brain was affected.

Strokes can be mild or severe. Afterwards a resident may experience any of the following:

- weakness or paralysis on one side of the body
- tendency to ignore a weak or paralyzed side of the body
- difficulty speaking or inability to speak
- difficulty understanding spoken or written words

- loss of sensations such as temperature or touch
- loss of bowel or bladder control
- confusion
- poor judgment
- memory loss
- loss of cognitive abilities
- difficulty swallowing

If the stroke was mild, the resident may experience few, if any, of these effects. Physical therapy may help stroke victims regain physical abilities. Speech and occupational therapy can also help a person learn to communicate and perform ADLs again.

GUIDELINES
Caring for Residents Recovering from Stroke

A resident with **hemiplegia**—paralysis on one side of the body, weakness, or loss of movement, will usually receive physical therapy or occupational therapy. Residents may also be instructed to perform leg exercises to improve circulation. Safety is always important when residents are exercising.

- Adapt procedures when providing personal care for residents with one-sided paralysis or weakness.

- When helping with transfers or walking, stand on the weaker side. Always use a gait belt for safety.

- Never refer to the weaker side as the "bad side," or talk about the "bad" leg or arm. Use the terms "weaker" or "involved" to refer to the side with paralysis.

- Residents with speech loss or communication problems may receive speech therapy. You may be asked to help. This may include helping residents recognize written words or spoken words. Speech therapists will also evaluate a resident's swallowing ability. They will decide if swallowing therapy or thickened liquids are needed.

🄱 Experiencing confusion or memory loss is upsetting. Residents often cry for no reason after suffering a stroke. Be very patient and understanding. Keeping a routine of care helps residents feel more secure.

Important ways nursing assistants help the resident recovering from stroke include

* Encourage independence and self-esteem. Let the resident do things for herself whenever possible even if you could do a better or faster job.

* Make tasks less difficult for the resident to do.

* Appreciate and acknowledge residents' efforts to do things for themselves even when they are unsuccessful.

* Praise even the smallest successes to build confidence.

GUIDELINES
Transferring a Resident with One-Sided Weakness

🄱 Support the weaker side.

🄱 Lead with the stronger side (Fig. 8-13).

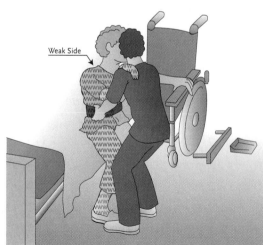

Weak Side

Fig. 8-13. When helping a resident transfer, support the weak side while leading with the stronger side.

GUIDELINES
Dressing a Resident with One-Sided Weakness

🄱 Dress weaker side first. Place the weaker arm or leg into the clothing first. This prevents unnecessary bending and stretching of the limb. Undress stronger side first. Lead with the stronger side. Then remove weaker arm or leg from clothing to prevent the limb from being stretched and twisted.

🄱 Provide adaptive equipment to help resident dress himself.

🄱 Encourage self-care.

GUIDELINES
Assisting a Resident with One-Sided Weakness with Eating

🄱 Place food in the resident's field of vision. They may have "blind spots." The nurse will determine a resident's field of vision (Fig. 8-14).

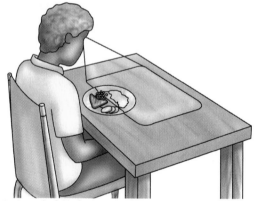

Fig. 8-14. The field of vision may be limited in a resident who has had a stroke. Be sure the resident can see what you place in front of him.

🄱 Use assistive devices such as utensils with built-up handle grips, plate guards, and drinking cups.

🄱 Watch for signs of choking.

🄱 Serve soft foods if swallowing is difficult.

🄱 Always place food in unaffected side of mouth.

🄱 Make sure food is swallowed before offering more bites.

GUIDELINES
Communicating with Residents Who Have Had a Stroke

Depending on the severity of the stroke and the degree of speech loss or confusion, the following tips may be helpful:

- Ⓖ Keep your questions and all directions simple.

- Ⓖ Phrase questions so they can be answered with a yes or no.

- Ⓖ Agree on signals, such as shaking or nodding the head, or raising a hand or finger to indicate yes or no

- Ⓖ Use pictures, gestures, or pointing to communicate. Use communication boards or special cards to make communication easier (Fig. 8-15).

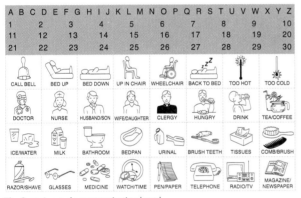

Fig. 8-15. A sample communication board.

- Ⓖ Use a pencil and paper if a resident is able to write. A thick handle or tape wrapped around it may help the resident hold it more easily.

- Ⓖ Keep the call signal within reach of residents. They can let you know when you are needed.

Ⓡ Never talk about residents as if they were not there. Just because they cannot speak does not mean they cannot hear. Speak to all residents with respect.

Head and Spinal Cord Injuries

Diving, sports injuries, and car and motorcycle accidents are common causes of these injuries. Head injuries can cause permanent brain damage. Spinal cord injuries depend on the force of impact and where the spine is injured. The higher the injury on the spinal cord, the greater the loss of function. People with head and spinal cord injuries may have **paraplegia**, or loss of function of lower body and legs. These injuries may also cause **quadriplegia**, in which the person is unable to use his legs, trunk, and arms (Fig. 8-16).

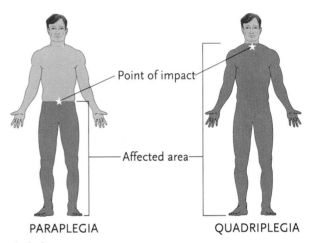

Fig. 8-16.

Help residents live as independently as possible. Residents need emotional support. Their specific needs will vary depending on the functions that have been lost and those that remain.

Unit 3: **Describe common diseases and disorders of the circulatory system**

High Blood Pressure (Hypertension)

When blood pressure consistently measures higher than 140/90, a person is diagnosed as having high blood pressure. High blood pressure, or hypertension, is caused by a hardening and narrowing of the blood vessels (Fig. 8-17). It can also result from kidney disease, tumors of the adrenal gland, complications of pregnancy, and head injury. High blood pressure can develop in persons of any age.

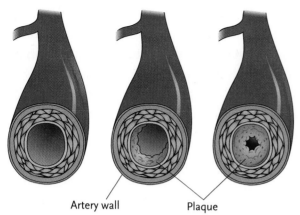

Fig. 8-17. Arteries may become hardened, or narrower, because of a buildup of plaque. Hardened arteries cause high blood pressure.

Signs and symptoms of high blood pressure are not always obvious, especially in the early stages of the disease. Often it is only discovered when a blood pressure measurement is taken in the doctor's office. Persons with the disease may complain of headache, blurred vision, and dizziness.

GUIDELINES
Caring for Residents with High Blood Pressure

- Because it can lead to serious problems such as CVA, heart attack, kidney disease, or blindness, treatment to control high blood pressure is essential. Residents may take medication that lowers cholesterol and reduce fluid in the body.

- They may also have a prescribed exercise program or be on a special low-fat, low-sodium diet.

Myocardial Infarction (MI) or Heart Attack

When blood flow to the heart muscle is completely blocked, oxygen and important nutrients fail to reach the cells in that region (Fig. 8-18). Waste products are not removed and the muscle cell dies. This is called a myocardial infarction or MI, or heart attack. See chapter 2 for warning signs of a heart attack.

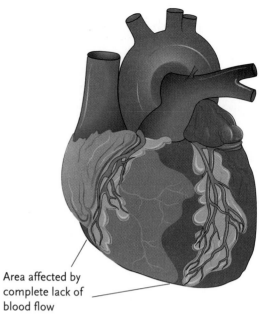

Area affected by complete lack of blood flow

Fig. 8-18. A heart attack occurs when blood flow to the heart or a portion of the heart is cut off completely.

GUIDELINES
Caring for Residents Recovering from Heart Attacks

- Generally residents will be placed on a regular exercise program.

- Residents may be on a diet that is low in fat and cholesterol and/or a low-sodium diet.

- Medications may be prescribed to regulate heart rate and blood pressure.

Coronary Artery Disease (CAD)

Coronary artery disease occurs when the blood vessels in the coronary arteries narrow. This reduces the supply of blood to the heart muscle and deprives it of oxygen and nutrients. Over time, as fatty deposits block the artery, the muscle that was supplied by the blood vessel dies. CAD can lead to heart attack or stroke.

The heart muscle that is not getting enough oxygen causes chest pain, or **angina pectoris**. Our heart needs more oxygen during exercise, stress, excitement, or a heavy meal.

In CAD, constricted blood vessels prevent the extra blood with oxygen from getting to the heart (Fig. 8-19).

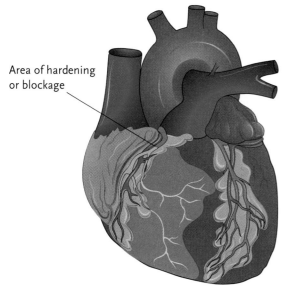

Area of hardening or blockage

Fig. 8-19. Angina pectoris results from the heart not getting enough oxygen.

The pain of angina pectoris is usually described as pressure or tightness in the left side of the chest or in the center behind the sternum or breastbone. Some people complain of the pain radiating or extending down the inside of the left arm or to the neck and left side of the jaw. A person suffering from angina pectoris may perspire or appear pale or grayish. The person may feel dizzy and have difficulty breathing.

GUIDELINES
Caring for Residents with Angina Pectoris

🅖 Rest is extremely important. Rest reduces the heart's need for extra oxygen. It helps the blood flow return to normal, often within three to fifteen minutes.

🅖 Medication is also necessary to relax the walls of the coronary arteries. This allows them to open and get more blood to the heart. This medication, nitroglycerin, is a small tablet that the resident places under the tongue. There it is dissolved and rapidly absorbed. Residents who have angina pectoris should keep nitroglycerin at hand to use as soon as

symptoms arise. Nursing assistants are not allowed to give any medication, including nitroglycerin. Inform the nurse if a resident needs help taking nitroglycerin. Nitroglycerin also is available as a patch. Do not remove the patch. Inform the nurse immediately if the patch comes off.

🅖 Residents may also be required to avoid heavy meals, overeating, intense exercise, and exposure to cold or hot and humid weather.

Congestive Heart Failure (CHF)

Coronary artery disease, heart attack, high blood pressure, or other disorders may all damage the heart. When the heart muscle has been severely damaged, the heart fails to pump effectively. Blood backs up into the heart instead of circulating. This is called CHF or congestive heart failure. It can occur on one or both sides of the heart.

OBSERVING AND REPORTING
CHF

⊕ difficulty breathing; coughing or gurgling with breathing

⊕ dizziness, confusion, and fainting

⊕ skin appears pale or blue

⊕ low blood pressure

⊕ swelling of the feet and ankles

⊕ bulging veins in the neck

⊕ weight gain from fluid retention

GUIDELINES
Caring for Residents with Congestive Heart Failure

🅖 Medications can strengthen the heart muscle and improve its pumping.

🅖 Medications help eliminate excess fluids. This means more frequent trips to the bathroom. Answer call lights promptly.

Common, Chronic, and Acute Conditions

⑤ A low-sodium diet may be recommended.

⑤ Intake of fluids and output of urine may need to be measured.

⑤ Resident must be weighed daily at the same time to note weight gain from fluid retention.

⑤ Elastic leg stockings may be applied to reduce swelling in feet and ankles. (See procedure below.)

⑤ Range of motion exercises improve muscle tone when activity and exercise are limited (Fig. 8-20). (See chapter 9 for range of motion information.)

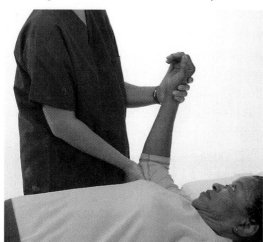

Fig. 8-20. Range of motion exercises improve muscle tone.

⑤ Assistance with personal care and ADLs may need to be provided.

Peripheral Vascular Disease (PVD)

Peripheral vascular disease is a condition in which the legs, feet, arms or hands do not have enough blood circulation. This is due to fatty deposits in the blood vessels that harden over time. Signs and symptoms include the following:

* cool arms and legs

* bluish nail beds from poor circulation

* swelling in hands or feet

* pale or bluish color to hands or feet

* ulcers of legs or feet

Some changes in a resident's health may lead to inactivity. A lack of ability to ambulate may contribute to PVD. For some cases of poor circulation to legs and feet, elastic stockings are ordered. These special stockings help prevent swelling and blood clots. They promote circulation. These stockings are called anti-embolic hose. Follow manufacturer's instructions and illustrations on how to put on stockings.

Putting a knee-high elastic stocking on resident

Equipment: elastic stockings

1. **Wash hands.**
   Provides for infection control.

2. **Identify yourself to resident by name. Address resident by name.**
   Resident has right to know identity of his or her caregiver. Addressing resident by name shows respect and establishes correct identification.

3. **Explain procedure to resident, speaking clearly, slowly, and directly, maintaining face-to-face contact whenever possible.**
   Promotes understanding and independence.

4. **Provide for resident's privacy during procedure with curtain, screen, or door.**
   Maintains resident's right to privacy and dignity.

5. **Turn stocking inside-out at least to heel area.**
   Allows stocking to roll on gently.

6. **Gently place foot of stocking over toes, foot, and heel (Fig. 8-21).**

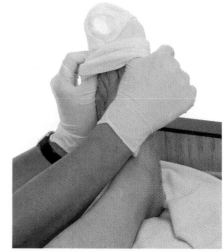

Fig. 8-21.

7. Gently pull top of stocking over foot, heel, and leg (Fig. 8-22).

Being gentle promotes resident's comfort and safety. Avoid force and over-extending joints.

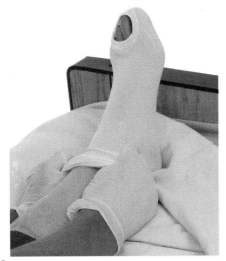

Fig. 8-22.

8. Make sure there are no twists or wrinkles in stocking after it is applied. It must fit smoothly.

Twists or wrinkles cause the stocking to be too tight, reducing circulation.

9. Before leaving resident, place signaling device within resident's reach.

Allows resident to communicate with staff as necessary.

10. Wash hands.

Provides for infection control.

11. Report any changes in resident to nurse.

Provides nurse with information to assess resident.

12. Document procedure according to facility guidelines.

What you write is a legal record of what you did. If you don't document it, legally it didn't happen.

👁 *You must place the stocking over toes and heel correctly. This makes it easier to bring it up the leg smoothly. Do not force the stocking over the foot.*

Unit 4: **Describe common diseases and disorders of the respiratory system**

Chronic Obstructive Pulmonary Disease (COPD)

COPD is a chronic disease. This means the resident may live for years with it but never be cured. Residents with COPD have difficulty breathing, especially in getting air out of the lungs. There are four chronic lung diseases that are grouped under COPD. They include:

- Chronic bronchitis
- Pulmonary emphysema
- Asthma
- Chronic bronchiectasis

Over time, a resident with any of these lung disorders becomes chronically ill and weakened. There is a high risk for acute lung infections, such as pneumonia. Pneumonia is an infection of the lungs. It is usually treated with antibiotics and other medications to reduce congestion and inflammation. Sometimes medications for lung conditions are given directly into the lungs by sprays or inhalers (Fig. 8-23).

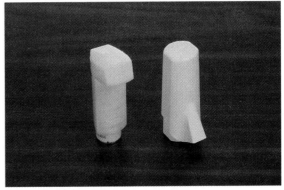

Fig. 8-23. An inhaler.

When the lungs and brain do not get enough oxygen, all body systems are affected. Residents may live with a constant fear of not being able to breathe. This can cause them to sit upright in an attempt to improve their ability to expand the lungs. These residents can have poor appetites. They usually do not get enough sleep. All of this can add to their feelings of weakness and poor health. They may feel they have lost control of their bodies, particularly with breathing. They may fear suffocation.

Residents with COPD may experience the following symptoms:

- chronic cough or wheeze
- difficulty breathing, especially with inhaling and exhaling deeply
- shortness of breath, especially during physical effort
- pale or cyanotic (blue) skin or reddish-purple skin
- mental confusion
- general state of weakness
- difficulty completing meals due to shortness of breath
- fear and anxiety

GUIDELINES
Caring for Residents with COPD:

🅖 Always observe and report signs of symptoms getting worse. Even colds or viruses can make residents very ill quickly.

🅖 Help residents sit upright or lean forward. Offer pillows to support them (Fig. 8-24).

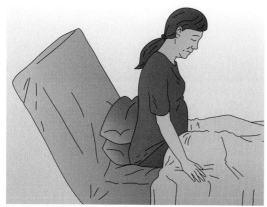

Fig. 8-24. It helps residents with COPD to sit upright and lean forward slightly.

🅖 Offer plenty of fluids and small frequent meals.

🅖 Encourage a well-balanced diet.

🅖 Keep oxygen supply available as ordered.

🅖 Be calm and supportive.

🅖 Use good infection control, especially with handwashing by the resident and the disposal of used tissues.

🅖 Encourage as much resident independence with ADLs as possible.

🅖 Remind residents to avoid situations where they may be exposed to infections, especially colds and the flu. Ensure that residents always have help available, especially in case of a breathing crisis.

🅖 Teach pursed-lip breathing. Pursed-lip breathing is placing the lips as if in a kiss and taking controlled breaths.

🅖 Encourage residents to save energy for important daily tasks. Encourage residents to rest during tasks.

OBSERVING AND REPORTING
COPD

- temperature over 101°F
- changes in breathing patterns, including shortness of breath
- changes in color or consistency of lung secretions
- changes in mental state or personality
- refusal to take medications as ordered
- excessive weight loss
- increasing dependence upon caregivers and family

Unit 5: Describe common diseases and disorders of the urinary system

Urinary Tract Infection (UTI)

UTIs cause inflammation of the bladder. This results in a painful burning feeling during urination. It also causes a frequent feeling of needing to urinate. UTIs may be caused by bacterial infection. Being confined to bed can cause urine to stay in the bladder too long. This helps bacteria to grow.

UTIs are more common in women. The urethra is much shorter in women than in men. This means bacteria can reach a woman's bladder more easily. To prevent UTIs, follow these guidelines:

- Encourage female residents to wipe from *front to back* after elimination (Fig. 8-25).

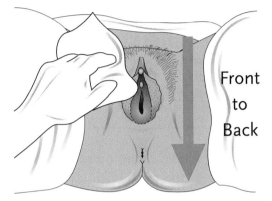

Fig. 8-25. After elimination, women need to wipe from front to back to prevent infection.

- Provide good perineal care when changing adult briefs.

- Encourage fluids.

- Offer bedpan or a trip to the toilet at least every two hours. Answer call lights promptly.

- Report cloudy urine or if a resident urinates often and in small quantities to the nurse.

Unit 6: **Describe common diseases and disorders of the gastrointestinal system**

Ostomy

An **ostomy** is the surgical removal of a portion of the intestines. It may be necessary due to bowel disease, cancer, or trauma. (More information on cancer is listed later in the chapter.) In a resident with an ostomy, the end of the intestine is brought out of the body through an artificial opening in the abdomen. This opening is called a **stoma**. Stool, or feces, are eliminated through the ostomy rather than through the anus.

The terms "colostomy" and "ileostomy" indicate what section of the intestine was removed and the type of stool that will be eliminated. In a colostomy, stool will generally be semi-solid. With an ileostomy, stool may be liquid and irritating to the resident's skin.

Residents who have had an ostomy wear a disposable bag that fits over the stoma to collect the feces (Fig. 8-26). The bag is attached to the skin by adhesive. Many people manage the ostomy appliance by themselves. If you are providing ostomy care, make certain the resident receives good skin care and hygiene. The ostomy bag should be emptied and cleaned or replaced whenever a stool is eliminated. Always wear gloves and wash hands carefully when providing ostomy care. Teach proper handwashing techniques to residents with ostomies.

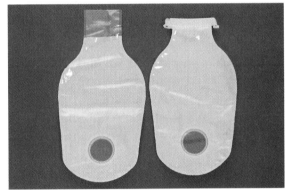

Fig. 8-26. An open and closed ostomy bag.

R *Many residents with ostomies feel they have lost control of a basic bodily function. They may be embarrassed or angry about the ostomy. Be sensitive and supportive when working with them. Always provide privacy for ostomy care.*

Caring for an ostomy

Equipment: bedpan, disposable bed protector, bath blanket, clean ostomy bag and belt/appliance, toilet paper, basin of warm water, soap or cleanser, washcloth, skin cream as ordered, two towels, plastic disposable bag, gloves

1. **Wash hands.**
   Provides for infection control.

2. **Identify yourself to resident by name. Address resident by name.**
   Resident has right to know identity of his or her caregiver. Addressing resident by name shows respect and establishes correct identification.

3. **Explain procedure to resident, speaking clearly, slowly, and directly, maintaining face-to-face contact whenever possible.**
   Promotes understanding and independence.

4. **Provide for resident's privacy during procedure with curtain, screen, or door.**
   Maintains resident's right to privacy and dignity.

5. **Adjust bed to a safe working level.**
   Prevents injury to you and to resident.

6. **Place protective sheet under resident. Cover resident with a bath blanket. Pull down the top sheet and blankets. Only expose ostomy site. Offer resident a towel to keep clothing dry.**
   Maintains resident's right to privacy and dignity.

7. **Put on gloves.**
   Provides for infection control.

8. **Remove ostomy bag carefully. Place it in plastic bag. Note the color, odor, consistency, and amount of stool in the bag.**
   Changes in stool can indicate a problem.

9. **Wipe the area around the stoma with toilet paper. Discard paper in plastic bag.**

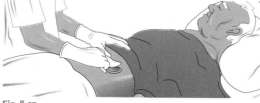

Fig. 8-27.

10. **Using a washcloth and warm soapy water, wash the area around the stoma. Pat dry with another towel. Apply cream as ordered.**
    Keeping skin clean and dry prevents skin breakdown.

11. **Place the clean ostomy appliance on resident. Make sure the bottom of the bag is clamped.**

12. **Remove disposable bed protector and discard. Place soiled linens in appropriate containers.**

13. **Remove bag and bedpan. Discard bag in proper container. Empty contents of bedpan into toilet.**

14. **Clean bedpan, pouring rinse water into toilet. Return to proper storage.**

15. **Remove and dispose of gloves properly.**

16. **Return bed to appropriate level. Place signaling device within resident's reach.**
    Lowering the bed provides for safety. Signaling device allows resident to communicate with staff as necessary.

17. **Wash hands.**
    Provides for infection control.

18. **Report any changes in resident to the nurse.**
    Provides nurse with information to assess resident.

19. **Document procedure according to facility guidelines.**
    What you write is a legal record of what you did. If you don't document it, legally it didn't happen.

Unit 7: Describe common diseases and disorders of the endocrine system

Diabetes

In **diabetes mellitus**, commonly called diabetes, the pancreas does not produce enough insulin. **Insulin** is needed to convert glucose, or natural sugar, into energy for the body. Without insulin to process glucose, these sugars collect in the blood. This causes problems with circulation and can damage vital organs. Diabetes commonly occurs in people with a family history of the illness, in the elderly, and among people who are obese. Two types of diabetes have been identified:

1. **Type I, or insulin-dependent diabetes mellitus (IDDM)**, is often called juvenile diabetes because it most often appears before age twenty. It will continue throughout a person's life. However, a person can develop Type I diabetes up to age 40. Type I diabetes is treated with insulin and a special diet.

2. **Type II, or noninsulin dependent diabetes mellitus (NIDDM)**, appears in adults. It can usually be controlled with diet and/or oral medications. This type is also called adult-

onset diabetes. Type II diabetes usually develops slowly. It is the milder form of diabetes mellitus. It typically develops after age 35. It often occurs in obese individuals or those with a family history of Type II.

People with diabetes mellitus may have the following signs and symptoms:

- increased thirst

- increased hunger

- weight loss

- elevated levels of blood sugar

- presence of sugar in the urine

- increased frequency of urination

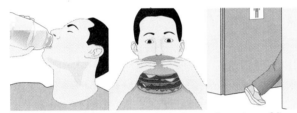

Fig. 8-28. Increased thirst, hunger, and urination are all symptoms of diabetes.

Diabetes can lead to the following problems:

- Changes in the circulatory system can cause heart attack and stroke, reduced circulation to the arms and legs, poor wound healing, and kidney and nerve damage.

- Damage to the eye can cause impaired vision and blindness.

- Poor circulation and impaired wound healing may result in leg and foot ulcers, infected wounds, and gangrene. Gangrene can lead to amputation.

- Insulin shock and diabetic coma can be life-threatening. See chapter 2 for more information on insulin shock and diabetic coma. Discuss each individual resident's status with your supervisor.

Encourage diabetic residents to wear comfortable, well-fitting shoes that do not hurt the feet. To avoid cuts or injuries to the feet, diabetics should never go barefoot. Cotton socks are best because they absorb sweat. Nursing assistants should never trim or clip a diabetic resident's toenails. Only a nurse or doctor should trim a diabetic's toenails.

People with diabetes must be very careful about what they eat. To keep their blood glucose levels near normal, they must eat the right amount of the right type of food at the right time. To make it easier to track what they should eat, diabetics often follow meal plans and use exchange lists.

A dietitian and resident will make up a meal plan that includes all the right types and amounts of food for each day. The resident uses exchange lists, or lists of similar foods that can substitute for one another, to make up a menu. For example, the meal plan might call for one starch and one fruit to be eaten as a snack. Looking at the exchange list, the resident may choose which starch and fruit he wants to eat. The equivalent serving size for each food is also given, so the person will get the right amount of carbohydrates, protein, and fat to meet the requirements. Using meal plans and exchange lists, a person with diabetes can control his diet while still making his own food choices.

Thoughtful care and careful observing and reporting are important. When working with residents with diabetes, follow care plan instructions and assignments to the letter.

GUIDELINES
Caring for Residents with Diabetes

- Follow diet instructions exactly. The intake of carbohydrates, including breads, potatoes, grains, pasta, and sugars, must be regulated. Meals must be eaten at the same time each day. The resident must eat everything that is served. If a resident refuses to eat what is served, or if you suspect that he or she is not following the diet, report this to the nurse.

- Ⓖ Encourage your resident to follow his exercise program. Regular exercise is important. It affects how quickly our bodies use the food we eat. Exercise also helps improve circulation. Exercises may include walking or other active exercise (Fig. 8-29).

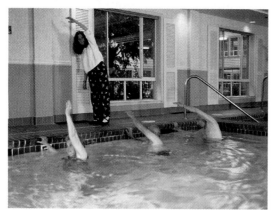

Fig. 8-29. Following an exercise program is very important for a diabetic resident.

- Ⓖ Observe the resident's management of insulin doses. Doses are calculated exactly. They will be given at the same time each day. Nursing assistants should know when residents take insulin and when their meals should be served. There always needs to be a balance between the insulin level and food intake.

Nursing assistants are sometimes assigned to perform urine and blood tests. Blood or urine tests determine sugar or insulin levels. However, not all states allow nursing assistants to do this. Know your state's rules. Perform tests only as directed (Fig. 8-30).

Perform foot care only as directed. Because poor circulation occurs in diabetics, even a small sore on the leg or foot can grow into a large wound. It can even result in amputation. Careful foot care, including regular prevention, is very important for diabetic residents. The goals of diabetic foot care are to check for signs of sores, to promote blood circulation, and to prevent infection.

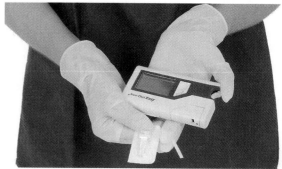

Fig. 8-30. This equipment measures glucose levels in the blood.

Unit 8: Describe common diseases and disorders of the reproductive system

Cancer of the reproductive organs is common. Older men often develop problems with the prostate gland. This can include enlargement or, sometimes, cancer. Either causes difficulty urinating and/or emptying the bladder. Surgery may be performed for cancer or to make the person more comfortable with elimination. Inform the nurse if you notice a weak urine stream or a lack of urination.

Elderly women have fewer reproductive problems. Some will have had reproductive organs surgically removed. Complaints of vaginal dryness are common and should be reported.

Unit 9: Describe common diseases and disorders of the lymphatic and immune systems

HIV and AIDS

Acquired immunodeficiency syndrome (AIDS) is an illness caused by the human immunodeficiency virus (HIV). HIV attacks the body's immune system and gradually disables it. Eventually the HIV-infected person has weakened resistance to other infections. Death is the result of these infections. However, medications help people live longer. HIV is a sexually transmitted disease. It is also spread through the blood, from infected needles, or to the fetus from its mother.

In general, HIV affects the body in stages. The first stage involves symptoms similar to flu, with fever, muscle aches, cough, and fatigue. These are symptoms of the body's immune system fighting the infection. As the infection worsens, the immune system overreacts and attacks not only the virus, but also normal tissue.

When the virus weakens the immune system in later stages, a cluster of problems may appear. These include infections, tumors, and central nervous system symptoms that would not occur if the immune system were healthy. This stage of the disease is known as AIDS.

In the late stages of AIDS, damage to the central nervous system may cause memory loss, poor coordination, paralysis, and confusion. These symptoms together are known as AIDS dementia complex.

The following are the signs and symptoms of HIV infection and AIDS:

- appetite loss
- involuntary weight loss of ten pounds or more
- vague, flu-like symptoms, including fever, cough, weakness, and severe or constant fatigue
- night sweats
- swollen lymph nodes in the neck, underarms, or groin
- excessive diarrhea
- dry cough
- skin rashes

- painful white spots in the mouth or on the tongue
- cold sores or fever blisters on the lips and flat, white ulcers on a reddened base in the mouth
- cauliflower-like warts on the skin and in the mouth
- inflamed and bleeding gums
- bruising that does not go away
- susceptibility to infection, particularly pneumonia, but also tuberculosis, herpes, bacterial infections, and hepatitis
- Kaposi's sarcoma, a form of skin cancer that appears as purple or red skin lesions (Fig. 8-31)
- AIDS dementia complex

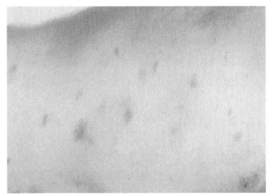

Fig. 8-31. A purple or red skin lesion called Kaposi's sarcoma can be a sign of AIDS.

Infections, such as pneumonia, tuberculosis, or hepatitis, invade the body because the immune system is weak and is unable to defend itself. These illnesses complicate AIDS. They further weaken the immune system. It is difficult to treat these infections because generally, over time, a person develops a resistance to some antibiotics. These infections are frequently the cause of death in people with AIDS.

Persons who are infected with HIV are treated with drugs that slow the progress of the disease, but do not cure it. The medicines must be taken at precise times. They have many unpleasant side effects. For some people, the medications work less well than for others. Other aspects of HIV treatment include relief of symptoms and prevention and treatment of infection. You can help prevent the spread of HIV/AIDS by carefully following standard precautions.

GUIDELINES
Caring for Residents with HIV/AIDS

- Involuntary weight loss occurs in almost all people who develop AIDS. High-protein and high-calorie meals can help maintain a healthy weight.

- Persons with poor immune systems are more sensitive to infections. Wash your hands often. Keep everything clean.

- Residents who have infections of the mouth may require food that is low in acid and neither cold nor hot. Spicy seasonings should be removed. Soft or pureed foods may be easier to swallow. Drinking liquid meals and fortified drinks may help ease the pain of chewing. Warm salt water or other rinses may help painful sores of the mouth. Good mouth care is essential.

- A person who has nausea or vomiting should eat small frequent meals, if possible. The person should eat slowly. Encourage fluids in between meals. These residents must maintain intake of fluids to balance lost fluids.

- Residents with mild diarrhea may require frequent small meals that are low in fat, fiber, and milk products. If diarrhea is severe, the resident's doctor may order a "BRAT" diet (a diet consisting of bananas, rice, apples, and toast). This diet is helpful for short-term use.

- Numbness, tingling, and pain in the feet and legs is usually treated with pain medications. Going without shoes or wearing loose, soft slippers may be helpful. If blankets cause pain, a bed cradle can be used to keep sheets and blankets from resting on legs and feet (Fig. 8-32).

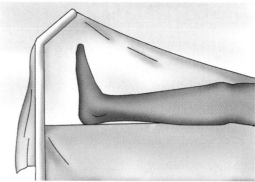

Fig. 8-32. A bed cradle keeps bed covers from pushing down on a resident's feet.

- Residents with HIV/AIDS may suffer from anxiety and depression. In addition, they often suffer the judgments of family, friends, and society. Some people blame them for their illness. People with HIV/AIDS may experience tremendous stress. They may feel uncertainty about their illness, health care, and finances. They may also have lost people in their social support network of friends and family.

- Residents with HIV/AIDS need support from others. This support may come from family, friends, religious and community groups, and support groups, as well as the healthcare team. Treat all your residents with respect. Help provide the emotional support they need.

- Withdrawal, avoidance of tasks, and mental slowness are symptoms that appear early in HIV infection. In addition, medications may cause side effects of this type. AIDS dementia complex may develop, causing further mental symptoms. There may also be muscle weakness and loss of muscle control, making falls a risk. Residents in this stage of the disease will need a safe environment and close supervision in their ADLs.

Cancer

Cancer is a general term used to describe many types of malignant tumors. A tumor is a cluster of abnormally growing cells. Benign tumors grow slowly in local areas. They are considered noncancerous. Malignant tumors grow rapidly and invade surrounding tissues.

Cancer invades local tissue, and it can spread to other parts of the body. Cancer can spread from the site where it first appeared and affect other body systems. In general, treatment is more difficult and cancer is more deadly after this has occurred. Cancer often appears first in the breast, colon, rectum, uterus, prostate, lungs, or skin.

Risk factors that appear to contribute to cancer include:

- tobacco use (Fig. 8-33)
- exposure to sunlight
- excessive alcohol intake
- chemicals and industrial agents
- food additives
- radiation
- poor nutrition
- lack of physical activity

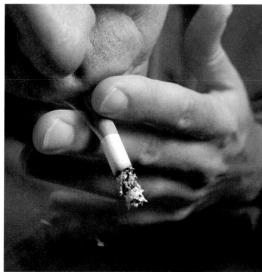

Fig. 8-33. Tobacco use is considered a risk for cancer.

When diagnosed early, cancer can often be treated and controlled. The American Cancer Society has identified seven warning signs of cancer. These are

Change in bowel or bladder habits

A sore that does not heal

Unusual bleeding or discharge from a body opening

Thickening or lump in the breast or elsewhere

Indigestion or difficulty swallowing

Obvious change in a wart or mole

Nagging cough or persistent hoarseness

People with cancer can often live longer and can sometimes recover if they are treated early. Treatments include

- surgery
- chemotherapy
- radiation (Fig. 8-34)

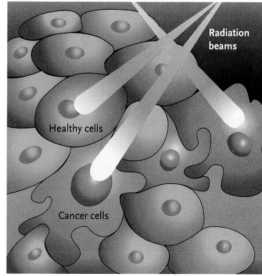

Fig. 8-34. Radiation is targeted at cancer cells, but it also destroys some healthy cells in its path.

GUIDELINES
Caring for Residents with Cancer

- **Each case is different.** Cancer is a general term and refers to many separate situations. Residents may expect to live many years or only several months. Treatment affects each person differently. Do not make assumptions about a resident's condition.

- ⑤ **Communication**. Residents may want to talk or may avoid talking. Respect each resident's needs. Be honest. Never tell a resident, "everything will be okay." Be sensitive. Remember that cancer is a disease, and we do not know its cause.

- ⑤ **Nutrition**. Good nutrition is extremely important for residents with cancer. Follow the care plan instructions and your assignments carefully. Use plastic utensils for a resident receiving chemotherapy. It makes food taste better. Silver utensils cause a bitter taste. Residents frequently have poor appetites. Encourage a variety of food.

- ⑤ **Pain control**. Cancer can cause terrible pain, especially in the late stages. Watch your resident for signs of pain and report them to the nurse.

- ⑤ **Skin care**. Use lotion regularly on dry or delicate skin. Do not apply lotion to areas receiving radiation therapy.

- ⑤ **Oral care**. Help residents brush and floss teeth regularly. Medications, nausea, vomiting, or mouth infections may cause a bad taste in the mouth.

- ⑤ **Self-image**. People with cancer may suffer from a low self-image because they are weak and their appearance has changed. For example, hair loss is a common side effect of chemotherapy. Be sensitive. Assist with grooming if desired.

- ⑤ **Psychosocial needs**. If visitors help cheer your resident, encourage them and do not intrude. If some times of day are better than others, suggest this.

- ⑤ **Family assistance**. Having a family member with cancer can be very difficult. Be alert to needs that are not being met or stresses created by the illness.

Many services and support groups are available for people with cancer and their families or caregivers. Hospitals, hospice programs, and religious organizations offer many resources. These include meal services, transportation to doctors' offices, counseling, and support groups. Check the local yellow pages under cancer, or call the local or state chapter of the American Cancer Society.

Unit 10: Describe mental illness, depression and related care

You first learned about mental health and mental illness in chapter 2. You can review the communication guidelines for mentally ill residents in that chapter.

There are many degrees of mental illness, from mild to severe. Clinical depression is a serious mental illness. It may cause intense mental, emotional, and physical pain, and disability.

Symptoms of clinical depression include the following:

- pain, including headaches, abdominal pain, and other body aches
- low energy or fatigue
- apathy, or lack of interest in activities
- irritability
- anxiety
- loss of appetite
- problems with sexual functioning and desire
- sleeplessness, difficulty sleeping, or excessive sleeping
- guilt
- difficulty concentrating
- repeated thoughts of suicide and death (Fig. 8-35)

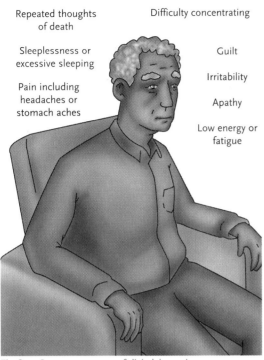

Repeated thoughts of death

Difficulty concentrating

Sleeplessness or excessive sleeping

Guilt

Irritability

Pain including headaches or stomach aches

Apathy

Low energy or fatigue

Fig. 8-35. Common symptoms of clinical depression.

- real or imagined physical symptoms
- events, situations, or people that seem to upset or excite residents

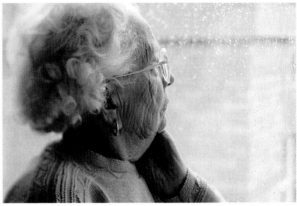

Fig. 8-36. Withdrawal is an important change to report.

GUIDELINES
Caring for Mentally Ill Residents

- Follow the care plan.
- Support the resident and family and friends.
- Maintain a professional attitude and be understanding with the family.
- Encourage residents to do as much for themselves as possible.

MENTALLY ILL RESIDENTS
Observing and Reporting

- changes in ability
- positive or negative mood changes, especially withdrawal (Fig. 8-36)
- behavior changes, including changes in personality, extreme behavior, and behavior that does not seem appropriate to the situation
- comments, even jokes, about hurting self or others
- failure to take medicine or improper use of medicine

NINE

Rehabilitation and Restorative Services

Unit 1: Describe the nursing assistant's role in rehabilitation

When a resident loses some ability to function due to illness or injury, rehabilitation services may be ordered. **Rehabilitation** is managed by professionals to restore a person to the highest possible level of functioning. These professionals include physical, occupational, and speech therapists. Rehabilitation involves all aspects of the person's disability. This includes psychological effects. The type of therapy used and how much progress is made are based on:

*   the type of illness or injury and how serious it is

*   the person's overall health

*   motivation of the resident and the rehabilitation team

*   when the rehabilitation process was begun

Restorative services usually follow rehabilitation. Their purpose is to keep the resident at the level achieved by the rehabilitation team. Restorative services also take a team approach. Staff create a care plan that includes the goals of restorative care. You will be an important member of this team. Nursing assistants spend more time with the residents than any other team member. Besides performing required tasks, remember to:

*   encourage the resident's independence

*   be supportive

*   be patient

RA *No matter what loss of function a resident has suffered, he or she has the right to expect staff to respond to his or her needs professionally—without judgment or bias.*

Unit 2: List ways to promote a resident's independence

Maintaining the resident's independence is a priority during and following rehabilitation and restorative services. When an active and independent person becomes dependent, physical and mental problems may result. The body becomes less mobile. The mind is less able to focus. Studies show that the more active a person stays, the better the mind and body function.

💜 *You will more easily understand physical and mental limitations that commonly occur as people age if you know the normal changes of aging.*

The staff's responsibility is to keep residents as active as possible—physically and mentally. **Ambulation** is walking. A resident who is ambulatory is one who can get out of bed and walk. Residents need to ambulate to maintain independence and prevent problems. Lack of mobility may result in a loss of the following:

*   independence
*   self-esteem
*   ability to move without help
*   muscle strength, leading to contractures
*   good circulation of blood

Regular ambulation and exercise help improve the following:

*   strength
*   sleep and relaxation
*   appetite
*   elimination
*   blood flow
*   oxygen level

Promoting a resident's social interactions and thinking abilities is important too. Most facilities have planned activities for residents that are geared to their ages and abilities. Social involvement should be encouraged. When possible, nursing assistants should participate in activities with residents. This promotes residents' independence. It also gives nursing assistants a chance to observe residents' abilities while they socialize.

📋 *The annual survey will look at the activities offered in the facility and see if all residents have an equal opportunity to participate.*

Unit 3: Describe assistive devices and equipment

Many devices are available to assist people who are recovering from or adapting to a physical condition. Examples are listed below and shown in Figure 9-1.

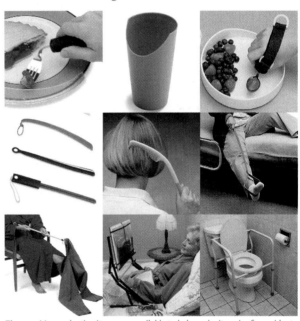

Fig. 9-1. Many adaptive items are available to help make it easier for residents to adapt to physical changes. (Photos courtesy of North Coast Medical, Inc., www.ncmedical.com, 800-821-9319)

*   Adaptive equipment is designed to assist the resident while doing ADLs. Each adaptive device is created to support a particular disability.
*   Personal care equipment includes long-handled brushes and combs.
*   Supportive devices are used when ambulating. Canes, walkers and crutches are examples.

- Safety devices, such as shower chairs and gait or transfer belts (Fig. 9-2), prevent accidents.

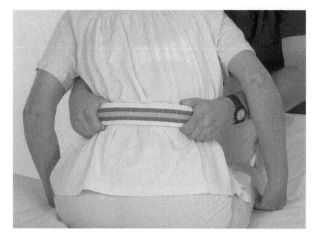

Fig. 9-2. A transfer belt, or gait belt, is used to assist residents who are able to walk but are weak or unsteady. The belt is made of canvas or other heavy material.

Check the care plan before helping a resident to ambulate. Discuss the resident's abilities and disabilities with the nurse. Know the resident's limitations and the goals for restoring and maintaining function. Any time you assist a resident, communicate what you would like to do. Allow him to do what he can do. The two of you will have to work together, especially during transfers.

Assisting a resident to ambulate

Equipment: transfer belt, non-skid shoes for the resident

1. **Wash hands.**
   Provides for infection control.

2. **Identify yourself to resident by name. Address resident by name.**
   Resident has right to know identity of his or her caregiver. Addressing resident by name shows respect and establishes correct identification.

3. **Explain procedure to resident, speaking clearly, slowly, and directly, maintaining face-to-face contact whenever possible.**
   Promotes understanding and independence.

4. **Provide for resident's privacy during procedure with curtain, screen, or door.**
   Maintains resident's right to privacy and dignity.

5. **Before ambulating, put on and properly fasten non-skid footwear on resident.**
   Promotes resident's safety. Prevents falls.

6. **Adjust bed to a safe working level, usually waist high.**
   Prevents injury to you and to resident.

7. **Stand in front of and face resident.**

8. **Brace resident's lower extremities. Bend your knees. Place one foot between resident's knees. If resident has a weak knee, brace it against your knee.**
   Promotes proper body mechanics. Reduces risk of back injury.

9. ***With transfer (gait) belt*: Place belt around resident's waist and grasp the belt, while assisting resident to stand.**

   ***Without transfer belt*: Place arms around resident's torso under resident's armpits, while assisting resident to stand.**

10. ***With transfer belt*: Walk slightly behind and to one side of resident for the full distance, while holding onto the transfer belt (Fig. 9-3).**

    ***Without transfer belt*: Walk slightly behind and to one side of resident for the full distance, with arm supporting resident's back.**

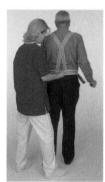

Fig. 9-3.

11. **After ambulation, remove transfer belt if used. Assist the resident to a comfortable position.**

12. **Return bed to appropriate level.**
    Lowering the bed promotes resident's safety.

13. **Before leaving resident, place signaling device within resident's reach.**
    Allows resident to communicate with staff as necessary.

14. **Wash hands.**
    Provides for infection control.

15. **Report any changes in resident to nurse.**
    Provides nurse with information to assess resident.

16. **Document procedure according to facility guidelines.**
    What you write is a legal record of what you did. If you don't document it, legally it didn't happen.

☀ *Before assisting with ambulation, you must apply non-skid footwear to the resident. It reduces the risk of the resident slipping and/or falling.*

Residents who have difficulty walking may use canes, walkers, or crutches to help themselves. Understanding the purpose of each device will help you know how to use it properly. The purpose of a cane is to help with balance. A straight cane is not designed to bear weight. A quad cane, with four rubber-tipped feet, is designed to bear a little weight (Fig. 9-4). Residents using canes should be able to bear weight on both legs. If one leg is weaker, the cane should be held in the hand on the strong side.

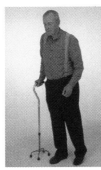

Fig. 9-4. A quad cane.

A walker is used when the resident can bear some weight on the legs. The walker provides excellent stability for residents who are unsteady or lack balance. The metal frame of the walker may have rubber-tipped feet and/or wheels. Crutches are used for residents who can bear no weight or limited weight on one leg. Some people use one crutch, and some use two.

When a resident uses a walker or cane, follow these guidelines. These guidelines will help keep the resident safe.

GUIDELINES
Cane or Walker Use

- Be sure the walker or cane is in good condition. It must have rubber tips on bottom. Walker may have wheels.

- If the walker has wheels, check them for safety.

- Be sure the resident is wearing non-skid shoes.

- Have the resident use the cane on his or her strong side.

- Have the resident use both hands on the walker.

- Stay near the person, on the weak side.

- Purses or clothing cannot hang on the walker.

- If height of the cane or walker does not seem to fit a resident, notify the nurse or physical therapist.

Assisting with ambulation for a resident using a cane, walker, or crutches

Equipment: transfer belt, non-skid shoes for resident, cane, walker, or crutches

1. **Wash hands.**
   Provides for infection control.

2. **Identify yourself to resident by name. Address resident by name.**
   Resident has right to know identity of his or her caregiver. Addressing resident by name shows respect and establishes correct identification.

3. **Explain procedure to resident, speaking clearly, slowly, and directly, maintaining face-to-face contact whenever possible.**
   Promotes understanding and independence.

4. **Provide for resident's privacy during procedure with curtain, screen, or door.**
   Maintains resident's right to privacy and dignity.

5. **Before ambulating, put on and properly fasten non-skid footwear on resident.**
   Promotes resident's safety. Prevents falls.

6. **Adjust bed to a safe working level, usually waist high.**
   Prevents injury to you and to resident.

7. **Stand in front of and face resident.**

8. **Brace resident's lower extremities. Bend your knees. Place one foot between resident's knees. If resident has a weak knee, brace it against your knee.**
   Promotes proper body mechanics. Reduces risk of back injury.

9. **Place transfer belt around resident's waist and grasp the belt, while assisting resident to stand.**
   Promotes resident's safety.

10. **Assist as necessary with ambulation.**

a. *Cane.* **Resident places cane about 12 inches in front of his stronger leg. He brings weaker leg even with cane. He then brings stronger leg forward slightly ahead of cane. Repeat (Fig. 9-5).**

b. *Walker.* Resident picks up or rolls the walker and places it about 12 inches in front of him. All four feet or wheels of the walker should be on the ground before resident steps forward to the walker. The walker should not be moved again until the resident has moved both feet forward and is in a steady position (Fig. 9-6). The resident should never put his feet ahead of the walker.
Promotes stability and prevents falls.

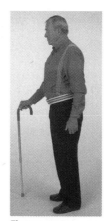
Fig. 9-5.

c. *Crutches.* Resident should be fitted for crutches and taught to use them correctly by a physical therapist or nurse. The resident may use the crutches several different ways, depending on what his weakness is. No matter how the resident is using the crutches, weight should be on the resident's hands and arms. Weight should not be on the underarm area (Fig. 9-7).

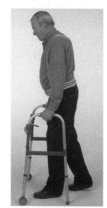
Fig. 9-6.

11. Walk slightly behind and to one side of resident. Hold the transfer belt if one is used.
Provides security.

12. Watch for obstacles in the resident's path. Encourage the resident to look ahead, rather than down at his or her feet.
Promotes resident's safety. Prevents injury.

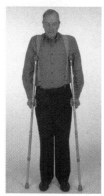
Fig. 9-7.

13. Encourage resident to rest if fatigued. Allowing a resident to become tired increases the chance of a fall. Let resident set the pace. Discuss how far he plans to go based on the physician's orders.
Prevents falls.

14. After ambulation, remove transfer belt. Assist resident to a position of comfort and safety.

15. Return bed to appropriate level.
Lowering the bed promotes resident's safety.

16. Before leaving resident, place signaling device within resident's reach.
Allows resident to communicate with staff as necessary.

17. Wash hands.
Provides for infection control.

18. Report any changes in resident to nurse.
Provides nurse with information to assess resident.

19. Document procedure according to facility guidelines.
What you write is a legal record of what you did. If you don't document it, legally it didn't happen.

👁 *You will be expected to promote residents' safety in all procedures you demonstrate.*

Unit 4: Describe positioning and how to assist with range of motion (ROM) exercises

Exercise helps people regain strength and mobility. It prevents disabilities from developing. People who are in bed for long periods of time are more likely to develop contractures. **Contractures** are the permanent and often painful stiffening of a joint and muscle. They are generally caused by immobility.

Residents who spend a lot of time in bed often need help getting into comfortable positions. They also need to change positions periodically. This helps avoid muscle stiffness and skin breakdown or pressure sores.

Bed-bound residents should be repositioned every two hours. This should be documented every time it is done.

Following are the five basic body positions:

1. **Supine** or lying flat on back (Fig. 9-8)

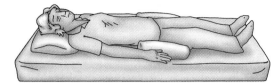

Fig. 9-8. A person in the supine position is lying flat on her back.

2. **Lateral** or side (Fig. 9-9)

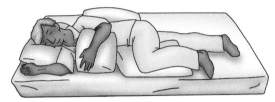

Fig. 9-9. A person in the lateral position is lying on his side.

3. **Prone** or lying on the stomach (Fig. 9-10)

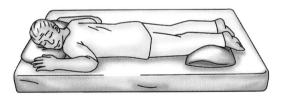

Fig. 9-10. A person in the prone position is lying on his stomach.

4. **Fowler's** or partially reclined (Fig. 9-11)

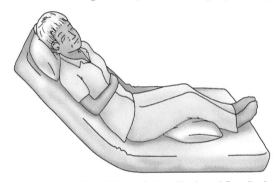

Fig. 9-11. A person lying in the Fowler's position is partially reclined.

5. **Sims'** or lying on the side with one leg drawn up (Fig. 9-12)

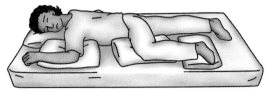

Fig. 9-12. A person lying in the Sims' position is lying on his side with one leg drawn up.

Residents who are confined to bed need to maintain good body alignment. This promotes recovery and prevents injury to muscles and joints. The following guidelines help residents maintain good alignment and make progress when they can get out of bed.

GUIDELINES
Alignment and Positioning

- Observe principles of alignment. Remember that proper alignment is based on straight lines. The spine should lie in a straight line. Pillows or rolled or folded blankets may be needed to support the small of the back and raise the knees or head in the supine position. They can support the head and one leg in the lateral position.

- Keep body parts in natural positions. In a natural hand position, the fingers are slightly curled. Use a rolled washcloth, gauze bandage, or a rubber ball inside the palm to support the fingers in this position (Fig. 9-13). Use footboards to keep covers from resting on feet in the supine position (Fig. 9-14).

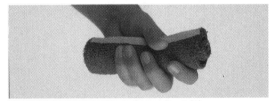

Fig. 9-13. Handrolls keep fingers from curling tightly.

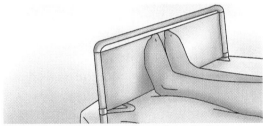

Fig. 9-14. Footboards keep covers from resting on the feet.

- Prevent external rotation of hips. When legs and hips are allowed to turn outward during long periods of bed rest, hip contractures can result. A rolled blanket or towel that is tucked along side the hip and thigh can prevent the leg from turning outward (Fig. 9-15).

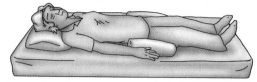

Fig. 9-15.

ⓖ Change positions frequently. Every two hours is usually adequate. Which positions a resident uses will depend on the resident's condition and preference. Check skin every time you reposition the resident.

ⓖ Have plenty of pillows available to provide support in the various positions.

ⓖ Use positioning devices (backrests, bed cradles and tables, footboards, and handrolls) (Fig. 9-16).

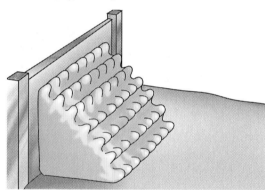

Fig. 9-16. A type of backrest.

ⓖ Give back rubs as ordered for comfort and relaxation.

Range of motion (ROM) exercises are exercises that put a particular joint through its full arc of motion. The purpose of range of motion exercises is to decrease or prevent contractures, improve strength, and increase circulation. When assisting with ROM exercises, the resident should not have any pain. If the resident complains of pain, stop the exercises. Report this to the nurse.

Passive range of motion (PROM) exercises are used when residents are not able to move on their own. When assisting with PROM exercises, support the resident's joints and move them through the range of motion. Active range of motion (AROM) exercises are performed by a resident himself. Your role in AROM exercises is to encourage the resident. Active assisted range of motion (AAROM) exercises are performed by the resident with some assistance and support from you.

You will never perform ROM exercises without a specific order from a doctor or physical therapist. When performing ROM exercises, begin at the resident's head and work down the body. You will move from upper extremities (arms) to the lower extremities (legs). These exercises are specific for each body area. They include the following movements:

- **Abduction**: moving a body part away from the body

- **Adduction**: moving a body part toward the body

- **Dorsiflexion**: bending backward

- **Rotation**: turning a joint

- **Extension**: straightening a body part

- **Flexion**: bending a body part

- **Pronation**: turning downward

- **Supination**: turning upward

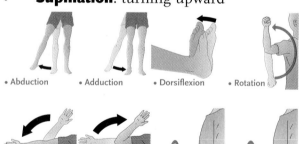

- Abduction   - Adduction   - Dorsiflexion   - Rotation

- Extension   - Flexion   - Pronation   - Supination

Fig. 9-17.

Assisting with passive range of motion (PROM) exercises

1.   **Wash hands.**
     Provides for infection control.

2.   **Identify yourself to resident by name. Address resident by name.**
     Resident has right to know identity of his or her caregiver. Addressing resident by name shows respect and establishes correct identification.

3.   **Explain procedure to resident, speaking clearly, slowly, and directly, maintaining face-to-face contact whenever possible.**
     Promotes understanding and independence.

4.   **Provide for resident's privacy during procedure with curtain, screen, or door.**
     Maintains resident's right to privacy and dignity.

5.   **Adjust bed to a safe working level, usually waist high.**
     Prevents injury to you and to resident.

6.   **Position the resident lying supine—flat on his or her back—on the bed. Position body in good alignment.**
     Reduces stress to joints.

7.   **Shoulder. Support resident's arm at elbow and wrist while performing ROM for shoulder. Place one hand above the elbow and the other hand around the wrist. Move the arm upward so that the upper arm is aligned with the side of the head (forward flexion) (Fig. 9-18).**

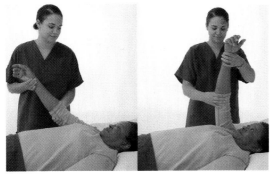

Fig. 9-18.

Move the arm downward to the side (extension) (Fig. 9-19).

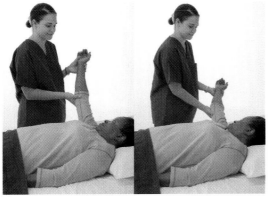

Fig. 9-19.

Bring the arm sideways away from the body to above the head (abduction) and back down (adduction) (Fig. 9-20).

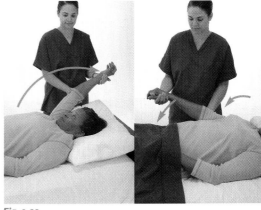

Fig. 9-20.

Bend the elbow and position it at the same level as the shoulder. Move the forearm down toward the body (internal rotation). Now move the forearm toward the head (external rotation) (Fig. 9-21).

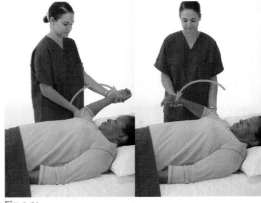

Fig. 9-21.

8.   **Elbow. Hold the resident's wrist with one hand, the elbow with the other hand. Bend the elbow so that the hand touches the shoulder on that same side (flexion). Straighten the arm (extension) (Fig. 9-22).**

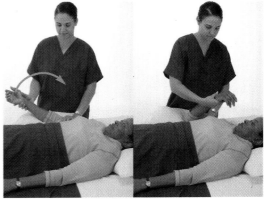

Fig. 9-22.

Rehabilitation and Restorative Services

Exercise the forearm by moving it so the palm is facing downward (pronation) and then the palm is facing upward (supination) (Fig. 9-23).

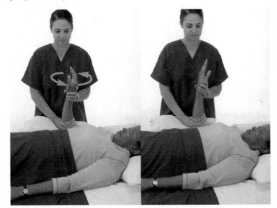

Fig. 9-23.

9. Wrist. Hold the wrist with one hand and use the fingers of the other hand to help the joint through the motions. Bend the hand down (flexion); bend the hand backwards (extension) (Fig. 9-24).

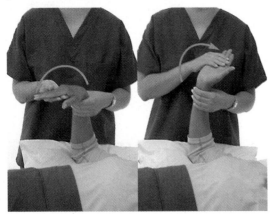

Fig. 9-24.

Turn the hand in the direction of the thumb (radial flexion). Then turn the hand in the direction of the little finger (ulnar flexion) (Fig. 9-25).

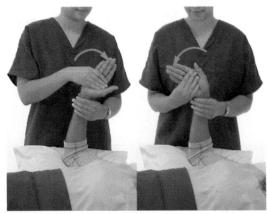

Fig. 9-25.

10. Thumb. Move the thumb away from the index finger (abduction). Move the thumb back next to the index finger (adduction) (Fig. 9-26).

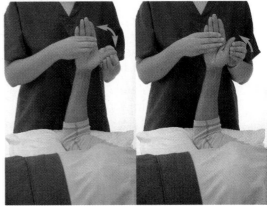

Fig. 9-26.

Touch each fingertip with the thumb (opposition) (Fig. 9-27).

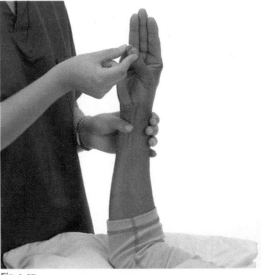

Fig. 9-27.

Bend thumb into the palm (flexion) and out to the side (extension) (Fig. 9-28).

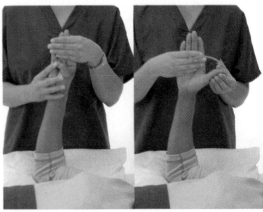

Fig. 9-28.

11. Fingers. Make the hand into a fist (flexion). Gently straighten out the fist (extension) (Fig. 9-29).

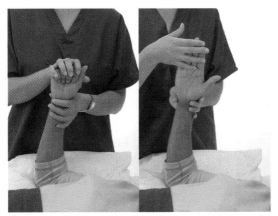

Fig. 9-29.

Spread the fingers and the thumb far apart from each other (abduction). Bring the fingers back next to each other (adduction) (Fig. 9-30).

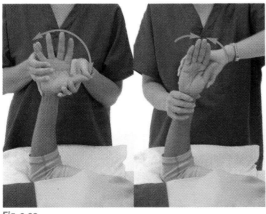

Fig. 9-30.

12. Hip. Support the leg by placing one hand under the knee and one under the ankle. Straighten the leg and raise it gently upward. Move the leg away from the other leg (abduction). Move the leg toward the other leg (adduction) (Fig. 9-31).

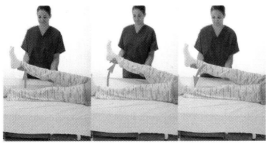

Fig. 9-31.

Gently turn the leg inward (internal rotation), then turn the leg outward (external rotation) (Fig. 9-32).

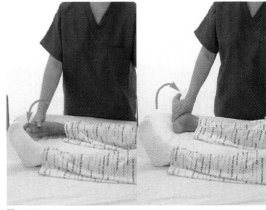

Fig. 9-32.

13. Knees. Bend the leg at the knee (flexion). Straighten the leg (extension) (Fig. 9-33).

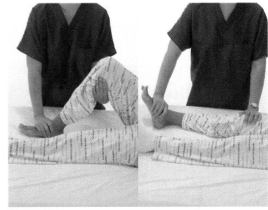

Fig. 9-33.

14. Ankles. Bend the foot up toward the leg (dorsiflexion). Turn the foot down away from the leg (plantar flexion) (Fig. 9-34).

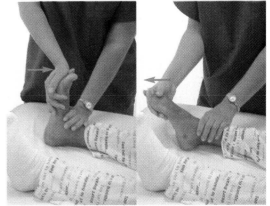

Fig. 9-34.

Rehabilitation and Restorative Services

Turn the inside of the foot inward toward the body (supination) and the sole of the foot so that it faces away from the body (pronation) (Fig. 9-35).

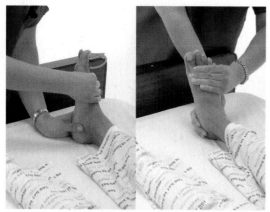

Fig. 9-35.

15. Toes. Curl and straighten the toes (flexion and extension) (Fig. 9-36).

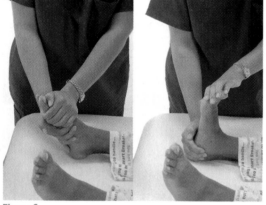

Fig. 9-36.

Gently spread the toes apart (abduction) (Fig. 9-37).

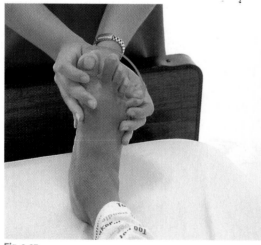

Fig. 9-37.

16. While supporting the limbs, move all joints gently, slowly, and smoothly through the range of motion to the point of resistance.

Stop exercises if any pain occurs.
Rapid movement may cause injury. Pain is a warning sign for injury.

17. Return bed to appropriate level.
Promotes resident's safety.

18. Before leaving resident, place signaling device within resident's reach.
Allows resident to communicate with staff as necessary.

19. Wash hands.
Provides for infection control.

20. Report any changes in resident to nurse.
Provides nurse with information to assess resident.

21. Document procedure according to facility guidelines.
What you write is a legal record of what you did. If you don't document it, legally it didn't happen.

☞ *When taking the certification exam, you may not be tested on ROM exercises for the entire body. You may only be tested on specific body parts. Regardless, it is important to remember that during ROM exercises, you must support the limbs at all times. Move joints gently and slowly. Always stop if pain occurs. Pain is a warning sign for injury.*

♥ *Note any decrease in range of motion or any pain experienced by the resident. If you find increased stiffness, notify the nurse. Resistance may be a sign that a contracture is developing.*

Unit 5: List guidelines for assisting with bowel and bladder retraining

Injury, illness, or inactivity may cause a loss of normal bowel or bladder function. Residents may need assistance in re-establishing a regular routine for going to the bathroom. Understand that problems with elimination can be embarrassing or difficult to talk about. Be sensitive to this.

Residents may experience incontinence. **Incontinence** is the inability to control the bowels or bladder. Always be professional when handling incontinence or assisting with re-establishing routines. Never show anger or frustration toward residents who are incontinent. Never refer to an incontinence brief or pad as a "diaper." Residents are not children, and this is disrespectful.

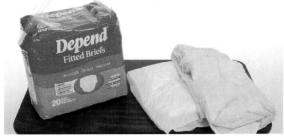

Fig. 9-38. A type of incontinence pad.

GUIDELINES
Bowel or Bladder Retraining

🅑 Follow standard precautions. Wear gloves when handling body wastes.

🅑 Follow the bowel and bladder training schedule carefully. Offer a commode or a trip to the bathroom before beginning long procedures (Fig. 9-39).

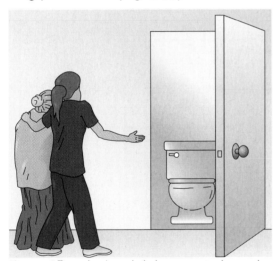

Fig. 9-39. Offer regular trips to the bathroom every two hours and as needed.

🅑 Explain the bowel or bladder training schedule to the resident.

🅑 Encourage residents to drink plenty of fluids. Do this even when urinary incontinence is a problem.

🅑 Encourage proper diet.

🅑 Answer call lights promptly. Residents cannot wait long when the urge to go to the bathroom occurs. Leave call lights within reach (Fig. 9-40).

🅑 Provide privacy for elimination—both in the bed and in the bathroom.

🅑 If the resident has difficulty urinating, try running the water in the sink. Have him or her lean forward slightly to put pressure on the bladder.

🅑 Never rush the resident.

🅑 Assist the resident with good perineal care. This prevents skin breakdown and promotes proper hygiene. Carefully observe for skin changes.

🅑 Discard wastes according to facility rules.

🅑 Discard clothing protectors and incontinence briefs properly. Some facilities require double bagging these items to stop odors from collecting.

🅑 Some facilities use washable bed pads or briefs. Follow standard precautions when rinsing prior to placing these items in the laundry.

🅑 Keep an accurate record of urination and bowel movements. This includes episodes of incontinence.

🅑 Offer positive words for successes.

When the resident is incontinent or cannot toilet when asked, be positive. Never make the resident feel like a failure. Words of praise and encouragement are essential for a successful program. Some residents will always be incontinent. Be patient. Offer these persons extra care and attention. Skin breakdown may lead to pressure sores without proper care. Always report changes in skin.

Rⓐ *Be professional when handling incontinence. It is hard enough for residents to handle incontinence without having to worry about your reactions. Showing frustration or anger is abusive behavior. Negative reactions only make the problem worse. Be patient with any setbacks that occur!*

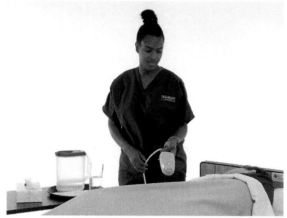

Fig. 9-40. Answer call lights promptly.

Unit 6: **Describe care and use of prosthetic devices**

A **prosthesis** is an artificial body part. It replaces a missing body part, such as an eye, arm, hand, foot or leg that has been amputated (surgically removed) due to injury or disease. The prosthesis will be custom-fitted to the resident (Fig. 9-41). When a body part has been amputated, the person's day-to day activities may be limited. A resident will need special attention to help him adjust to these changes. When the condition is new and a prosthesis has been ordered, a physical and/or occupational therapist may work with the resident.

You will assist the resident with ADLs and ambulation. You must know how to care for the limb and how to use a prosthesis. Prostheses are expensive. Take great care when handling them.

GUIDELINES
Care of a Prosthesis

- Follow the care plan regarding the care of the prosthesis and the limb.

- A nurse or therapist will demonstrate application of a prosthesis. Follow instructions on applying and removing the prosthesis. Follow the manufacturer's directions for care.

- Keep the prosthesis and the skin under it dry and clean.

- If ordered, apply a stump sock before putting on the prosthesis

- Never try to repair a prosthesis. Report any problems with it to the nurse

- Observe the skin on the stump and report any redness or open areas.

- Never display negative feelings regarding the stump during care.

- If the resident has an artificial eye, review the care plan with the nurse. Know any special instructions for assisting the resident with care.

- Again, take care with prostheses. They are very expensive.

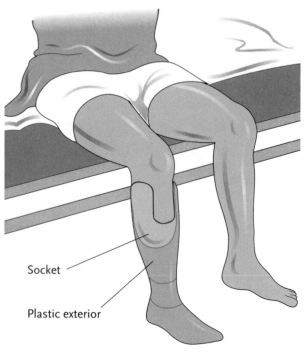

Socket

Plastic exterior

Fig. 9-41. Prostheses are specially fitted, expensive pieces of equipment.

TEN

Caring for Yourself

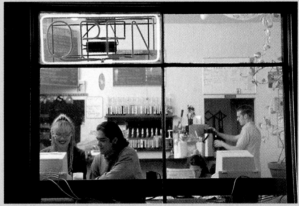

Fig. 10-1. Searching the Internet is one good way to find a job.

Unit 1: **Describe how to find a great job**

If you are in a school program, you may soon be looking for a job. To find a job, you must first find potential employers. Then you must contact them to find out about job opportunities. To find potential employers, use the newspaper, the telephone book, the Internet, or personal contacts (Fig. 10-1). Ask your instructor about potential employers. Some schools maintain a list of employers seeking nursing assistants.

Once you have a good list of potential employers, you need to contact them about job opportunities. Phoning first is a good way to learn what jobs are available and how to apply with each potential employer.

When making an appointment, ask what information to bring with you. Make sure you have this information with you when you go. Some of these documents may include the following:

- Identification: driver's license, social security card, birth certificate, passport, or other official form of identification to prove who you are

- Proof of your legal status in this country and proof that you are legally able to work, even if you're a U.S.-born citizen. All employers must have files showing that all employees are legally allowed to work in this country. Do not be offended by this request.

- High school diploma or equivalency, school transcripts, and diploma or certificate from your nursing assistant training course. It is a good idea to have your instructor's name and phone number, too.

- References are people who can be called to recommend you as an employee. They can include former employers, former teachers, your minister, or your doctor. Do not use relatives or friends as references. You can ask your references beforehand to write general letters for you, addressed "To whom it may concern," explaining how they know you and describing your skills, qualities, and habits. Take copies of these with you for employers to keep.

On one sheet of paper, write down the general information you will need to complete an application. Take it with you. This will save time and avoid mistakes.

Include the following general information:

- your address and phone number

- your birth date

- your social security number

- the name and address of the school or program where you were trained and the date you completed your training, as well as certification numbers and expiration dates from a nursing assistant certification card, if you have one

- the names, titles, addresses, and phone numbers of your previous employers, and the dates you worked there

- the names and phone numbers of your references

- the days and hours you are available to work

- a brief statement of why you are chang-

ing jobs or why you want to work as a nursing assistant

Fill out the application carefully and neatly. Never lie on a job application. Before you write anything, read it all the way through once. If you do not understand what is being asked, find out before filling in that space.

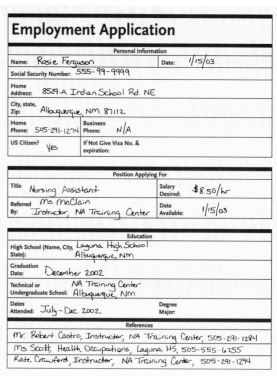

Fig. 10-2. A sample job application.

By law, your employer must perform a criminal background check. You may be asked to sign a form granting the facility permission to do this. Do not take it personally; it is a law intended to protect residents.

To make the best impression at a job interview, behave professionally:

- Dress neatly and appropriately.

- Shower or bathe, and use deodorant.

- Wear only simple makeup and jewelry or none at all.

- Arrive ten or fifteen minutes early.

- Introduce yourself, smile, and shake hands (Fig. 10-3).

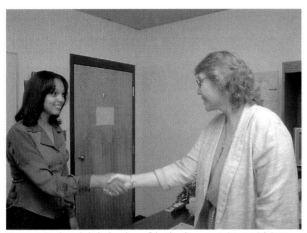

Fig. 10-3. Smile and shake hands confidently when you arrive at a job interview.

- Answer all questions clearly and completely.

- Make eye contact to show you are sincere (Fig. 10-4).

- Avoid using slang words or expressions.

- Never eat, drink, chew gum, or smoke in an interview.

- Sit up or stand up straight, and look happy to be there.

- Do not bring friends or children to the interview with you.

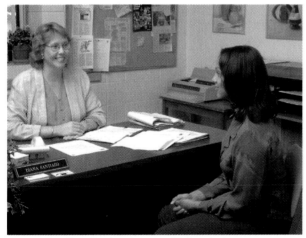

Fig. 10-4. Be polite and make eye contact while interviewing.

Be positive when answering any questions the interviewer asks. Emphasize what you enjoy or think you will enjoy about being a nursing assistant. Do not complain about any previous jobs you held. Make it clear that you are hardworking and willing to work with all kinds of residents.

Usually interviewers will ask if you have any questions. Have some prepared and written down so you do not forget things you really want to know. Questions you may want to ask include the following:

- What hours would I work?

- What benefits does the job include? Is health insurance available? Would I get paid sick days or holidays?

- What orientation or training will be provided?

- How much contact would I have with my supervisor?

- How soon will you be making a decision about this position?

Later in the interview, you may want to ask about salary or wages if you have not already been told what it would be.

Unit 2: **Describe ways to be a great employee**

Handling criticism is difficult for most of us. Being able to accept criticism and learn from it is important in all relationships, including employment. From time to time you will receive evaluations from your employer. These evaluations contain ideas to help you improve your job performance. Here are some ideas for handling criticism and using it to your benefit:

- Listen to the message that is being sent. Do not get so upset that you are unable to really understand the message.

- Hostile criticism and constructive criticism are not the same. Hostile criticism is angry and negative. Examples are "You are useless!" or "You are lazy and slow." Hostile criticism should not come from your employer or supervisor. You may experience hostile criticism from residents, family members,

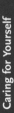

or others. The best response is to say something like "I'm sorry you are so disappointed," and nothing more. Give the person a chance to calm down before trying to discuss their comments.

- Constructive criticism may come from your employer, supervisor, or others. Constructive criticism is intended to help you improve. An example is: "You really need to be on time more often. Please make more of an effort to do so." Listening to and acting on constructive criticism can help you be more successful in your job, so pay attention to it. (Fig. 10-5).

- If you are not sure how to avoid a mistake you have made, always ask the person criticizing you for suggestions in improving your performance.

- Apologize and move on. If you have made a mistake, apologize as needed. This may be to your supervisor, your resident, or others. Learn what you can from the incident and put it behind you. Do not dwell on it or hold a grudge. Being able to respond professionally to criticism is important for success in any job.

If you decide to change jobs, be responsible. Always give your employer at least two weeks' written notice that you will be leaving. Otherwise, your facility may be understaffed and both the residents and other nursing assistants will suffer. In addition, future employers may talk with past supervisors. People who change jobs too often or who do not give notice before leaving are less likely to be hired.

Unit 3: Review guidelines for behaving professionally on the job

Be professional in your new job! This will help you keep your job. It will also help you

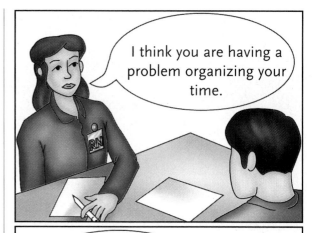

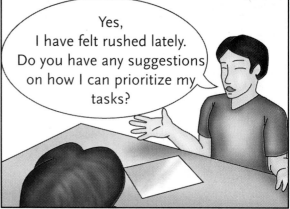

Fig. 10-5. Ask for suggestions when receiving constructive criticism.

earn the respect of co-workers and residents. Remember to

- Be responsible; always call in if you cannot show up for a scheduled work shift.

- Be on time for your shift.

- Be clean and neatly dressed and groomed (Fig. 10-6).

- Maintain a positive attitude.

- Follow policies and procedures.

- Document and report carefully and correctly.

- Ask questions when you do not know or understand something.

- Communicate with residents and members of the healthcare team.

- Report anything that keeps you from completing duties.

- Offer positive suggestions for improving care.

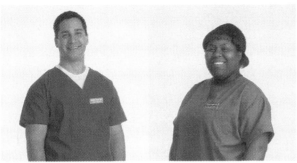

Fig. 10-6. Being clean and well groomed is an important part of being a nursing assistant.

Unit 4: **Describe continuing education for nursing assistants**

In the United States, each state maintains a registry for certified nursing assistants (CNAs). Each state has slightly different requirements for maintaining certification. Learn your requirements and follow them exactly or you will not be able to keep working as a nursing assistant. Ask your instructor or employer for the requirements in your state. You should know how many hours of in-service education are required per year. Also know how long an absence from working as a nursing assistant is allowed without losing your certification. You may need to work a certain number of hours in a long-term care facility to remain on the registry.

The federal government requires nursing assistants to have 12 hours of continuing education each year. Some states may require more. In-service continuing education courses help you keep your knowledge and skills fresh. Classes also provide new information about conditions, challenges that you face in working with residents, or regulation changes.

Your employer may be responsible for offering in-service courses, but you are responsible for successfully attending and completing them. It is your responsibility to obey education requirements. Specifically, you must do the following:

- sign up for the course or find out where it is offered

- attend all class sessions

- pay attention and complete all the class requirements

- make the most of your time during in-service programs. PARTICIPATE! (Fig. 10-7)

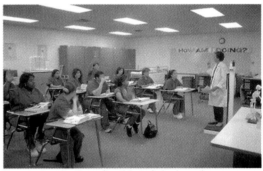

Fig. 10-7. Pay attention and participate during in-service courses.

- keep original copies of all certificates and records of your successful attendance so you can prove you took the class

📋 *The annual survey includes a review of personnel files to assure that all state and federal education, training, certification, and employee health regulations are met.*

Unit 5: **Define stress and discuss ways to manage it**

Stress is the state of being frightened, excited, confused, in danger, or irritated. We usually think only bad things cause stress. However, positive situations cause stress too. For example, getting married or having a new baby are usually positive situations. But both can bring enormous stress from the changes they bring to our lives.

You may be thrilled when you get a new job as a nursing assistant, but starting work may also cause you stress. You may be afraid of making mistakes, excited about earning money or helping people, or confused about how to perform your new duties. Learning how to recognize stress and what causes it is helpful. Then you can master a few simple techniques for relaxing and learn to manage stress.

A **stressor** is something that causes stress. Anything can be a stressor if it causes you stress. Some examples include

- divorce
- marriage
- a new baby
- children leaving home
- feeling unprepared for a task
- losing a job
- starting a new job
- problems at work
- new responsibilities at work
- supervisors
- co-workers
- residents
- illness
- finances

Stress is not only an emotional response. It is also a physical response. When we experience stress, certain changes occur in our bodies. The endocrine system may produce more of the hormone adrenaline. This can increase nervous system response, heart rate, respiratory rate, and blood pressure. This is why, in stressful situations, your heart beats fast, you breathe hard, and you feel warm or perspire.

Each of us has a different tolerance level for stress. In other words, what one person would find overwhelming might not bother another person. Your tolerance of stress depends on your personality, life experiences, and physical health.

GUIDELINES
Managing Stress

To manage the stress in your life, develop healthy habits of diet, exercise, and lifestyle.

- Eat nutritious foods.
- Exercise regularly (Fig. 10-8).
- Get enough sleep.
- Drink only in moderation.
- Do not smoke.

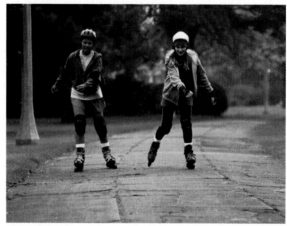

Fig. 10-8. Regular exercise is one healthy way to decrease stress.

Find time at least a few times a week to do something relaxing, such as taking a walk, reading a book, or sewing.

Not managing stress can cause many problems. Some of these problems will affect how well you do your job. Signs that you are not managing stress include the following:

- showing anger or being abusive toward residents
- arguing with your supervisor about assignments
- having poor relationships with co-workers and residents
- complaining about your job and your responsibilities
- feeling work-related burn-out
- feeling tired even when you are rested
- having a difficult time focusing on residents and procedures

RA *You may never hit a resident, **no matter what**. If you feel out of control, seek help, advice, or at least put some distance between you and the situation.*

Stress can seem overwhelming when you try to handle it yourself. Often just talking about stress or stressors can help you manage it better. Sometimes another person can offer helpful suggestions. Or, you may think of new ways to handle stress just by talking it through with another person.

Obtain help from one or more of the following when managing stress:

- your supervisor or another member of the care team for work-related stress

- your family

- your friends

- your church, synagogue, mosque, or temple

- your physician

- a local mental health agency

- any phone hotline that deals with related problems (check your local yellow pages)

It is not appropriate to talk to your residents or their family members about your personal or job-related stress.

One of the best ways of managing stress in your life is to develop a plan for managing stress. The plan can include nice things you will do for yourself every day and things to do in stressful situations. When you think about a plan, you first need to answer the following questions:

- What are the sources of stress in my life?

- When do I most often feel stress?

- What effects of stress do I see in my life?

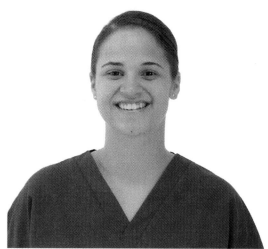

Fig. 10-9. Do something nice for yourself every day to help manage stress.

- What can I change to decrease the stress I feel?

- What do I have to learn to cope with because I cannot change it?

When you have answered these questions, you will have a clearer picture of the challenges you face. Then you can come up with strategies for managing stress.

Sometimes a relaxation exercise can help you feel refreshed and relaxed in only a short time. The following is a simple relaxation exercise. Try it out and see if it helps you feel more relaxed.

The body scan.
1. *Close your eyes.*
2. *Pay attention to your breathing and posture.*
3. *Be sure you are comfortable.*
4. *Starting at the balls of your feet, concentrate on your feet.*
5. *Discover any tension hidden in the feet and try to relax and release the tension.*
6. *Continue very slowly.*
7. *Take a breath between each body part.*
8. *Move up from the feet, focusing on and relaxing the legs, knees, thighs, hips, stomach, back, shoulders, neck, jaw, eyes, forehead, and scalp.*
9. *Take a few very deep breaths and open your eyes.*

Caring for Yourself

Look back over all you have learned in this program. Your work as a nursing assistant is very important. Every day may be different and challenging. In a hundred ways every week you will offer help that only a caring person like you can provide.

Do not forget to value the work you have chosen to do. It is important. Sometimes your work can mean the difference between living with independence and dignity versus living without. The difference you make is sometimes life versus death. Look in the face of each of your residents and know that you are doing important work. Look in a mirror when you get home. Be proud of how you make your living (Fig. 10-10).

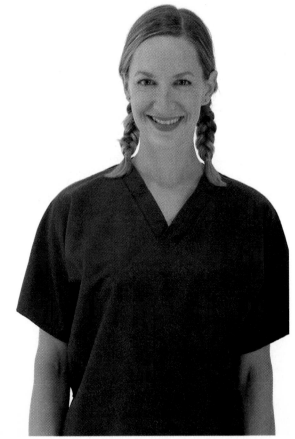

Fig. 10-10.

COMMON ABBREVIATIONS

a	before
ADL	activities of daily living
am, AM	morning, before noon
amb	ambulatory
amt	amount
ap	apical
approx.	approximately
ax.	axillary (armpit)
b.i.d.	two times a day
BM	bowel movement
BP, B/P	blood pressure
BRP	bathroom privileges
c̄	with
cath	catheter
cc	cubic centimeters
CHF	congestive heart failure
CNA	certified nursing assistant
c/o	complains of
COPD	chronic obstructive pulmonary disorder
CPR	cardiopulmonary resuscitation
CVA	cerebrovascular accident, stroke
DNR	do not resuscitate
DON	director of nursing
dx	diagnosis
E.R.	emergency room
exam	examination
FF	force fluids
f. (fl.)	fluid
ft	foot
h, hr	hour
H_2O	water

HBV	hepatitis B virus
HIV	human immunodeficiency virus
hs	hour of sleep
ht	height
hyper	above normal, too fast, rapid
hypo	low, less than normal
hs	hour of sleep
ht	height
I&O	intake and output
inc	incontinent
IV	intravenous (within vein)
isol	isolation
lab	laboratory
lb.	pound
LPN	Licensed Practical Nurse
LTC	long-term care
LVN	Licensed Vocational Nurse
meds	medications
min	minute
ml	milliliter
mm Hg	millimeters of mercury
MRSA	methicillin resistant staph aureus
N/A	not applicable
N.A.	nursing assistant
NPO	nothing by mouth
O_2	oxygen
OBRA	Omnibus Budget Reconciliation Act
OOB	out of bed
oz	ounce
p	after
peri care	perineal care

PPE	personal protective equipment
p.r.n., prn	when necessary
q2h, q3h, etc.	every 2 hours, every 3 hours, and so on
q.d.	every day
q.h.	every hour
q.i.d., qid	four times a day
q.o.d.	every other day
R	respirations
reg.	regular
rehab	rehabilitation
RN	Registered Nurse
ROM	range of motion
rt.	right
s̄	without
stat	immediately
spec.	specimen
STD	sexually transmitted disease
std. prec.	standard precautions
T.	temperature
TB	tuberculosis
temp	temperature
t.i.d., tid	three times a day
T.P.R.	temperature, pulse, and respiration
U/A	urinalysis
URI	upper respiratory infection
UTI	urinary tract infection
vs	vital signs
w/c	wheelchair
wt.	weight

INDEX